THEATRE NURSING

THEATRE NURSING
A guide for students and trainees

Ann Adams BA (Hons), SRN

Heinemann Nursing

Heinemann Nursing
An imprint of Heinemann Professional Publishing Ltd
Halley Court, Jordan Hill, Oxford OX2 8EJ

OXFORD   LONDON   SINGAPORE   NAIROBI   IBADAN   KINGSTON

First published 1990

British Library Cataloguing in Publication Data
Adams, Ann
Theatre Nursing.
1. Hospitals, Operating theatres, Nursing
I. Title

610.73'677

ISBN 0 433 00074 0

Typeset by Lasertext Ltd, Thomas Street, Stretford, Manchester M32 0JT
Printed in Great Britain by Biddles Ltd., Guildford and Kings Lynn.

Contents

Preface

This book has been written for those encountering the enigmatic world of the operating department for the first time.

Its aim is to give a simple introduction to the new environment, equipment and procedures and to show how the principles of patient centred care are practised here. Primarily, emphasis has been placed on giving a detailed description of the role of the theatre nurse in each area. Much of this information, however, is also directly relevant to allied professionals, and in particular trainee operating department assistants. Thus the book provides a model for any novice in the department.

There is a balance between sound clinical material for immediate reference and more thought provoking matter for discussion. The book also addresses itself to identifying the unique skills which can be learnt in the department, which will enhance the performance of every trained nurse in any setting.

Above all, the book aims to give orientation and to dispel any sense of mystery.

Ann Adams

Acknowledgements

I have to thank many people for their help and support in the preparation of this book. In particular, I want to thank Alan Bidwell, Theatre Manager, Guy's Hospital, London; Caroline Bedford, Theatre Manager, The Sussex Clinic, Hastings, and Gay Moncur, Theatre Manager at The Royal Free Hospital, London, who generously gave their time in reading and constructively criticizing the text.

I should also like to thank my late husband Simon for his encouragement, and my parents and mother-in-law for much babysitting.

1

Introduction:
this strange world

My first view of this strange world was as a student nurse. My room in the nurses' home overlooked the back of the surgical wards, where four operating theatres were visible, piled one on top of the other. But my inquisitive gaze was frustrated by heavily frosted windows, refracting the bright lights and blurring shapes. All that was visible was a world of dimly lit figures, moving to and fro; mere shadows illuminated by enormous saucers of light. I was fascinated.

Placements on surgical wards increased my curiosity. What did happen to patients once they went through those swing doors with the peculiar porthole windows? What strange rituals took place inside? The odd chances I had to peer through the portholes – when the anaesthetist wasn't looking and the patient I had accompanied was accommodatingly drowsy – gave me no clearer idea. My curiosity was not to be satisfied for almost 3 years, until I was finally allocated to work in the gynaecological theatre for 10 weeks. That time has proved to be one of my happiest training memories.

I know, however, that not every learner nurse feels as I did, and that initial contact with this new environment can be very daunting. Richard Gordon's memory of his first visit to the operating theatre expresses well what most of us feel:

> I pushed open the theatre door and stepped inside reverently, like a tourist entering a cathedral. Standing by the door, my hands clasped tightly behind me, all I wanted was completely to escape notice. I felt that even my breathing, which sounded in my ears like the bellows of a church organ, would disturb the sterile noiseless efficiency of the place (Gordon, 1961).

Ridiculously and uncomfortably garbed, we are intruders entering the sacred place of an alien sect. Fearful in this awesome atmosphere, we are aware of nothing save our own potential to cause havoc and our desire to blend into the well scrubbed, gleaming, bare expanses of wall. Wearing hat and mask we cannot hear what is said to us, but suspect we are being told: 'Don't touch that!' or : 'Watch where you are walking!' Nor can anyone hear what we say to them. Altogether we feel alienated, useless, unable to contribute anything. The best strategy seems to be to remain still and quiet, hoping we will be overlooked. What are the rules that govern this place? How are we to apply the learnt principles of patient-centred care in this coldly clinical environment? It really is a very strange world.

As one who has perpetrated the mysteries of this department, I am writing this book in an effort to dispel the feelings of alienation and uselessness. I aim to show that beneath the hats, masks and gowns are theatre nurses, whose concerns and priorities are the same as those of nurses working elsewhere in the hospital; namely, to give a very high standard of patient care.

Four thoughts were uppermost in my mind whilst I was writing. The first was to address myself to the sense of disorientation common to learner nurses on first entering the department. 'What shall I do?' and 'What should I be doing?' are familiar cries. I hope that by giving very detailed outlines of the role of the learner nurse in each area of the department – anaesthetics, in the theatre itself, and in recovery – to have confronted and alleviated this negative feeling.

My second thought was to aim for simplicity in both language and explanation. I have tried to keep the book as free from jargon as possible, and I hope that the explanations regarding equipment and procedures are clear and easy to follow.

Thirdly, I wanted to achieve a balance between providing a sound clinical background for learners, with chapters that can be used for immediate reference in the practical situation, such as *Instruments* and *Sutures and wound closure* as well as more thought-provoking matter. Chapters such as *Getting the most from your theatre allocation* and *Operating department nursing as a career* debate topical issues surrounding the work, and could be used as catalysts for discussion in tutorial sessions.

Above all, I hope to have communicated my own enthusiasm for theatre nursing, and to dispel any doubts students may harbour about the place of nurses in this department (see Chapter 15). I have taken great pains to point out the very real and unique assets the department possesses, and in Chapter 14 learners are confronted with the task of evaluating this for themselves. My hope is that students will leave the department armed with new skills and insight into the world of the theatre nurse, which will enhance their contribution to society as a trained nurse, in whatever specialty they choose to pursue.

Reference

Gordon, R. (1961). *Doctor in the House*. London: Penguin, p. 64.

2

The physical environment

Perhaps the best way to start looking at this new department is to empty the busy landscape of people. This will give a clearer view of the layout and basic equipment.

THEATRE DESIGN

The prevention of wound infection is the most important consideration when designing an operating department. It needs to be the very cleanest part of the hospital – self-contained and away from the general hospital traffic. Isolation has the added benefit of peace and quiet, reducing stress levels for both patients and staff. If prevention of infection is the most important consideration, the safety of patients and staff ranks a close second. These two topics will be referred to many times in subsequent chapters.

Today most operating theatres are grouped together to form a *department*, which also comprises rest rooms, changing rooms, teaching, storage and reception areas. This compactness allows for a better use of resources and facilities, including the skills of trained theatre personnel. An operating *suite* is one functioning unit of a department: an anaesthetic room, clean preparation room, scrub-up area, operating theatre, sluice room and exit bay.

By the end of your operating department allocation you will have a highly developed sense of the meaning of the words clean and dirty. Bearing in mind our major preoccupation, the prevention of wound infection, all journeys within the department are made from clean to dirty areas, never the other way round. Let us consider the progress of some important people and things.

Patients enter the department from the hospital corridor via a transfer bay. Here they are usually lifted on to a theatre trolley, leaving the ward bed outside. Next they enter either a holding area or else move directly to the anaesthetic room. Finally they enter the theatre itself where surgery is to be performed. The journey has been one through progressively cleaner areas, arriving finally at the cleanest of all.

Once the wound has been closed and covered with dressing, it is safe for the patient to return to the ward via progressively more dirty areas: through the exit bay, recovery and the hospital corridor. There are also psychological benefits in moving patients constantly in one direction. Those arriving for surgery are not confronted by the sight of immediately postoperative patients going to recovery. Nor are they troubled by seeing soiled instruments or used suction bottles leaving the suite from the previous operation. These could ruin the good effects of careful preoperative preparation and premedication.

Instruments and equipment are brought from outside the department into clean store rooms. Instruments are often supplied in pre-packed sterilized trays by the Theatre Sterile Supplies Unit (TSSU); these trays may be taken and opened in the clean preparation room. Alternatively, instruments are sterilized here. Finally, they enter the theatre ready for use on the scrub nurse's trolley. At the end of an operation, dirty instruments, linen and rubbish are removed to the sluice room, and when correctly packaged for disposal, to agreed collection points. Porters then take them via a dirty corridor to their several destinations: the TSSU, laundry or hospital incinerator.

Theatre personnel follow the same clean to dirty rule. They enter the department via a changing room where outdoor clothing is left. Once attired in correct theatre dress they can proceed to a suite along a clean corridor. Here they enter via the clean preparation room or the scrub-area, and like the patient, leave through the exit bay.

Such movement, from clean to dirty areas, will be second nature to you after a while. You will understand why you cannot take rubbish out of the theatre through the clean preparation room, and why the trained staff throw up their hands in horror when a new medical student takes a specimen out to the scrub-up sink for dissection! Following the clean to dirty rule is essential if cross-infection is to be prevented.

To maintain the highest possible standards of cleanliness, care must be taken in choosing *floor and wall coverings*. The material of which they are made must be able to withstand continued washing with detergent without any surface deterioration. There must also be as few places as possible where dust can gather; hence the preference for featureless walls. You may also have noticed that there are no sharp corners anywhere. These will all have been rounded off, again for the same reason, so as not to harbour dust and for easy cleaning. These considerations coupled with the need for brighter lights throughout the department create the dreary starkness of which many complain. Unrelieved expanses of bare gleaming walls with little to break up the monotony depress some students, but you can appreciate that this is a case where patient safety has to come first.

Another important consideration when choosing floor and wall coverings is the need to prevent explosions caused by sparks of static electricity. Many inflammable substances and a large quantity of electrical equipment are kept in operating departments (these hazards will be discussed more fully later) so all flooring and the soles of staff footwear must be made of an anti-static material. Every department is also well equipped with fire-fighting appliances, alarms, exits and a detailed procedure to follow in the event of fire.

Ventilation

The direction of air flow in the operating department follows the same direction as all other people and things: from clean to dirty areas. Air is sucked in from the roof, passes through a filter where it is cleaned, humidified and the temperature regulated before being circulated in the department by high-level diffusers in the walls and ceilings. To ensure the cleanest air for the cleanest areas, that circulated in the theatre and clean preparation room is at the highest pressure. Air therefore flows outwards to less clean areas; the pressure prevents any back-flow. Each theatre suite is ventilated in this manner, which means that there is no mixing of air between them and the risk of cross-infection is minimized. For the system to work well an enclosed area is necessary. This is one reason why you should remember to keep as many doors closed as possible, and why the flow of traffic in theatres should be kept to a minimum.

You may come across more specialized types of ventilation, such as the *laminar flow* system. Here, filtered air is diffused in horizontal planes in one direction only, without any turbulence. You might also see a *Charnley – Howarth tent*, which is a tent inside the theatre made from panels of a heavy, transparent plastic material. Air is pumped in and sucked out of the tent at an exceedingly high pressure, giving as many as up to 300 air changes per hour.

These specialized types of ventilation are used mainly for orthopaedic or ophthalmic surgery, where the prevention of joint or intraocular infection is vital. These two areas have very little resistance to infection introduced by trauma or surgery, due to their lack of blood supply. Prophylactic antibiotic cover is normally given during the operative procedure, as infection here can be very debilitating and difficult to treat.

THE ANAESTHETIC ROOM

The mechanics of anaesthesia will be dealt with fully in Chapter 5, but while the suite is empty of people let's take a look at three important pieces of equipment – the anaesthetic machine, suction apparatus and the drug cupboard.

The anaesthetic machine

This probably looks to you a very complicated piece of equipment with all its cylinders, bottles and tubing (Fig. 2.1), but in reality it is very simple. It is a means of delivering to the patient a mixture of anaesthetic gases and volatile agents in the form of vapours.

Let us look at its salient features one by one. On the side of the machine are cylinders of the different gases, each with a pressure gauge on top. At the top left-hand corner are the flowmeters or rotameters. When the cylinders are open these are used to regulate the flow of the gases, measured in litres per minute. Next to them is a vaporizer. This contains the volatile anaesthetic agent to be mixed with the gases. As the gases flow through the vaporizer, this agent evaporates, and thus it is carried on through the circuit. The dial on the top of the vaporizer controls the percentage of saturation of the gases by the agent. This mixture is then inhaled by the patient via the black anti-static corrugated rubber tubing, often known as elephant tubing! On the bottom of the machine is a ventilator. If the patient is not breathing spontaneously – if the respiratory muscles have been paralysed by an anaesthetic drug – this machine will inflate the lungs artificially. The rate and depth of respiration can again be regulated.

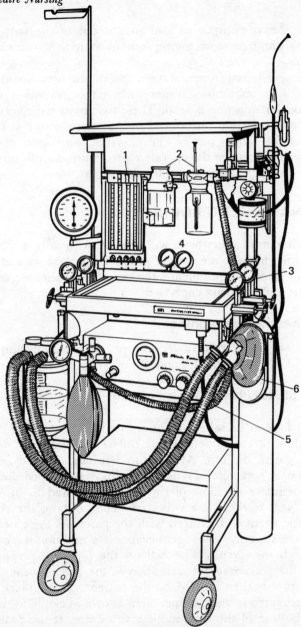

Fig. 2.1 The anaesthetic machine. **1** Rotameter or flowmeter. **2** Vaporizer. **3** Cylinder supply gauge. **4** Pipeline gas supply gauges. **5** Ventilator. **6** Combined anaesthetic tubing carrying mixture of gases and volatile agents to the patient

Many additions can be made to this basic apparatus: commonly there is a sphygmomanometer, a suction unit and equipment to monitor blood pressure, pulse and respirations. You will no doubt come across other additions, but remember that they are all extra to the basic functioning machine. The reality is not as complex as it may at first appear.

Suction apparatus

Suction apparatus is vital in an anaesthetic room. Under anaesthesia patients are not always able to clear their own airway, so an artificial means of doing this must always be at hand. If there is not a suction unit attached to the anaesthetic machine, then there will be one mounted on the wall or else attached to a yellow suction pipe hanging down from the ceiling. Failing that there will be a portable electric suction machine. This is one piece of equipment which you should locate as soon as you come to work in the anaesthetic room.

The units are simple to operate. Once the yellow suction pipe is plugged in at the wall or ceiling, a handle on the side will switch them on. The strength of suction can be modified to low, medium, or high by a separate control. Disposable plastic tubing and Yankaur suction heads are attached to an outlet in the lid of the bottle. These must be changed for each patient. The bottles are easy to take apart for washing or sterilizing as necessary. Do take care to test the function of the unit once it is reassembled however, as poorly connected bottles and tubing will not function adequately. The electric suction machines work in the same manner. Once plugged into the mains they are operated by a simple on/off switch, with an extra control to increase or decrease the suction. Again the bottles are easily taken apart.

The drug cupboard

The drug cupboard for the suite is usually located in the anaesthetic room, as it is here that the majority of drugs are given. As on the wards you will find a mixture of scheduled and some controlled drugs kept here. The same hospital policies for storage, ordering and record-keeping are adhered to. A member of the trained nursing team will always hold the keys.

Before leaving the anaesthetic room there is one more feature to notice at this point. If the suite is modern or has been recently up-graded, there may be *piped gases* in your anaesthetic room. If so, these will be used instead of the cylinders on the anaesthetic machine, which then become a back-up supply should the piped source fail. The pipes hang down from the ceiling together with the yellow suction pipe in a bundle of four. The white pipe carries oxygen (O_2), the blue one nitrous oxide (N_2O) and the grey one compressed air. The colours conform to the British Standard code. The pipes are plugged into the back of the anaesthetic machine for use.

These are the main features worth noting when you are new to the department. The rest of the anaesthetic equipment will be dealt with in Chapter 5.

THE OPERATING THEATRE

This is a far more sparsely furnished room for the reasons of cleanliness already discussed. The centre piece of the room is the *operating table* (Fig. 2.2). The table has a metal base and a cushioned, black anti-static rubber mattress. It is on wheels, so that once the brake at the foot of the table is released, it is fully mobile. The table can also be made higher or lower. This is usually controlled by a projecting foot pedal near the base, unless your department is lucky enough to possess an electric table.

The operating table is a very versatile piece of equipment. It has to be in order to accommodate the great variety of different operating positions. As well as the above features, it is also equipped with gears to tilt or 'break' it into different shapes, levers to tilt its extremities, and a whole range of attachable and detachable accessories. The detachable parts will be discussed first.

The head and leg sections of the table can both be removed. This is done by pressing a release button on the side of the adjacent section, and pulling. This frees the two prongs holding the end section in place, allowing it to be removed. Two people are normally required to do this – one to press the button and one to pull – as all parts of the table are extremely heavy. Let us now also deal with the levers, as these are features of the two detachable ends, found on the underside. By using these, the head and leg ends can be raised above or tipped below the horizontal plane of the table on a ratchet. To achieve one of these positions,

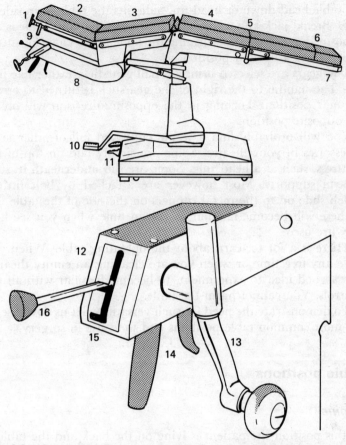

Fig. 2.2 Operating table of the 'break' type. **Inset** details of the control arm. **1** Fine adjustment control. **2** Head section. **3** Upper trunk section. **4** Lower trunk section. **5** Perineal recess. **6** Detachable leg section. **7** Leg section control. **8** Control arm (see inset). **9** Quick release control. **10** Height control pedal. **11** Three position brake pedal. **12** Gear lever position for Trendelenburg movement. **13** Main control handle. **14** Pistol grip handles to adjust control arm position. **15** Gear lever position for lateral movement. **16** Gear lever engaging chair and break movement

the lever must be pulled upwards, the end section moved to the desired angle and then the lever released. This locks the table into the new position.

Now the gears. These are located on one side of the table, towards the head end. There are three gears to choose from: Trendelenburg, side, and 'break' or chair. Trendelenburg tips the table head-down or head-up. Side tilts the table from side to side. 'Break' jack-knifes the table in the middle, and chair is the opposite movement, transforming the table into a chair for sitting patients in an upright position.

The gears are selected using a small gearstick, rather like in a car. The handle to the right of the gearstick is turned to create the new position. Turning in the opposite direction will create the opposite position.

You will probably find a whole cupboard full of other table accessories in your theatre. Some are simply laid on top of the mattress, such as a head ring. Some are slid underneath it, such as arm supports. Most however are attached by bolt fittings which slide on to the metal runners on the side of the table. All of these will become familiar to you in time when you see how they are used.

There is a lot to learn about the operating table. When you have any free time or when you are cleaning an empty theatre, it is a good idea to experiment, to become familiar with all the controls. You cannot harm the table.

To demonstrate the need for such versatility, let us now discuss the most common table positions and their use in surgery.

Table positions

Supine

In this position the patient is lying on the back and the table is horizontal. Accessories to be added are supports for the arms to prevent them falling over the edges of the table, which could result in damage to the brachial plexus of nerves, and heel supports to prevent the formation of pressure sores. This is the most common surgical position, used largely for abdominal work, but also for a wide range of other specialties.

Prone

The opposite of supine is prone. The patient lies on the front and the table is horizontal. The head end of the table may be removed and a horseshoe-shaped facial support substituted. Pillows should be placed on top of the mattress to give support under the chest and pelvis. The knees and feet may also need some padding where

they come into contact with the table, and again arm supports
will be needed. This position is used mainly for spinal surgery
and in general surgery for excision of a pilonidal sinus.

Trendelenburg

Trendelenburg is a position in which the patient is lying flat on
the back with the table tipped head downwards. The same
accessories as for the supine position are needed. This position
was originally designed for operating on varicose veins as it
aids venous drainage, but today it is most commonly used in
gynaecological surgery. The position allows good access to the
pelvic organs, as gravity causes the intestines to drop away from
the operative field.

Reverse Trendelenburg

As you might expect, this is its opposite. The patient lies flat on
the back with the table tilted head upwards. This position is used
for operations on the head and neck. In addition to the supports
for the supine position, a head ring and a sandbag under the
shoulders may be used to allow the surgeon better access.

Lithotomy

This is the 'legs up' position used for perineal operations. Special
lithotomy poles with stirrups to support the patient's feet are
bolted on to the distal end of the table and the leg section is
removed. Arm supports are still needed (Fig. 2.3). Care must be
taken to lift both legs simultaneously into the stirrups, otherwise
damage may be sustained to the hip and sacroiliac joints.

Kidney position

As its name suggests, this gives the best surgical access to the
kidneys. The patient lies on the side and the table is broken in
the middle. A back support and Carter–Braine arm support are
needed; both bolt on to the table. A stomach support or strapping
across the body may also be added to increase the stability of the
position. The patient's lower leg is flexed at the knee and a pillow
is used as a pad between the legs, usually at knee level. Ankles
and heels will also need support.

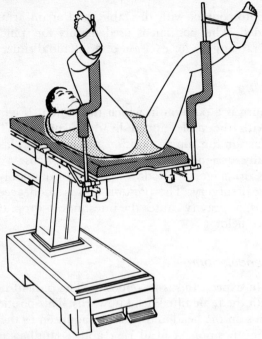

Fig. 2.3 Lithotomy position

'Chair' position

This is rarely used, but it is mentioned here for completeness. The table is broken in the opposite direction to the kidney position. Foot and arm supports are added together with the horsehoe-shaped facial support. Neurosurgeons use this position for posterior fossa surgery.

Moving on to another prominent piece of equipment, the *diathermy machine* – this is an electrical machine which gives the surgeon power to perform two functions: to coagulate bleeding blood vessels and to incise tissue. Power to do this – the electric current – is transferred from the machine via a diathermy lead connected to the surgeon's diathermy forceps (both of these are found among the sterilized instruments for each operation). The power is released by using the diathermy pedals: the blue one for coagulation and the yellow one for cutting. The strength of the current passed is modified by two numbered controls, one for each function (see Fig. 2.4).

Passing an electric current through a patient's body puts him

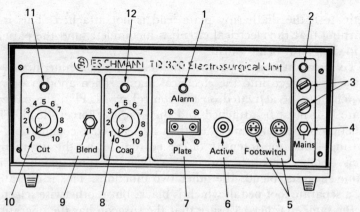

Fig. 2.4 Diathermy machine. **1** Alarm indicator lamp for plate safety (red). **2** Mains (power) pilot lamp (green). **3** Live and neutral fuseholders. **4** Mains on/off (I/O) switch. **5** Footswitch sockets. **6** Fingerswitch/active cable socket. **7** Patient plate electrode socket. **8** Coagulation output control. **9** Blend on/off (I/O) switch. **10** Cutting output control. **11** Cut pilot lamp (yellow). **12** Coagulation pilot lamp (blue)

or her at risk of sustaining electrical burns. In order to make the procedure safe, the live electrode – the surgeon's forceps – must be balanced by an indifferent electrode to pass the current back to the diathermy machine. This then forms a complete electrical circuit. The diathermy plate fulfils this role. It is a wide, flexible metal plate, which can be adhered to the skin or else supported by a crêpe bandage or Velcro band. For complete safety, the plate must have good contact with a large area of dry skin. If the plate becomes wrinkled it is useless, which is why a fresh one must be used for each patient. Some of the plates on the market do not guarantee complete safety from burns unless the skin to which it is adhered has been shaved: check the manufacturer's instructions. For adults the plate is normally fixed to the thigh, but for children, under the buttocks will give a larger area of skin contact. Finally, you should check that the patient is in contact with no other metal, such as a drip stand or lithotomy pole, as these areas of contact could give rise to diathermy burns.

The diathermy plate is also attached to the diathermy machine by a lead. This lead does not need to be sterile and the shape of its connection is entirely different to that of the lead attached to the live electrode (forceps). It is therefore impossible for any mix-ups to occur. All machines have an alarm system which will activate if the diathermy plate lead is not attached. This is a warning that the electrical circuit is incomplete, and the patient is in danger of being burnt.

To recap on how to operate the diathermy machine, firstly, it must be plugged into the electrical mains. Then another on/off switch must be activated on the control panel. First the patient plate lead must be attached and then the live forceps lead. The function of the machine must then be selected – coagulation or cutting – and the intensity of the current set by the numbered dials. (Some machines also have a 'blend' setting which, as its name suggests, blends the other two functions. This is operated by a separate foot pedal, which is black, but is otherwise selected in the same manner.) Ensure that the surgeon has the operating pedals at his or her feet, and that they are correctly attached to the machine. If at any time the alarm should sound, the diathermy machine must not be used until the patient is safely earthed.

You may come across a *bipolar diathermy* machine in your suite. This performs the same functions as conventional diathermy, but eliminates some of the risks. Both the live and indifferent electrodes are incorporated in the surgeon's forceps, so that the electrical current travels back down the same lead, making the circuit much more compact. The patient therefore does not need a diathermy plate.

Suction apparatus is found in the operating theatre also. Not only is it used by the anaesthetist for clearing an airway, but also by the surgical team for evacuating blood and other fluids from the operating field. Some suction units are incorporated into the diathermy machine, while in other suites separate appliances, operated by the yellow suction pipes of the type already described, are in use. Whereas one suction bottle is adequate in the anaesthetic room, at least two are required in the theatre, as larger volumes of aspirate are encountered during surgery. You will need to locate the switch which transfers the suction power to the second bottle, enabling you to detach and empty the first. Another feature to note is the gradations on the side of the bottle, for measuring the amount of aspirate. It is important to know how much blood has been lost during an operation.

Operating lights

There are usually two operating lights in a theatre; these may be two of the same size or one large one and a small satellite. They may be attached to the ceiling at one fixed point on a flexible boom, so that they have a circular range of movement, or else mounted in a groove, allowing them to be moved up and down its length. The rounded heads of the lights can also be tilted; the larger ones have a metal bar around them to make this easier. The lights are easily manoeuvred, which again is necessary to accommodate the needs of surgery. Good lighting is needed to carry out an operation, and lighting a wound from two converging angles is designed to eliminate shadows. You should also notice the focusing switch on the side of the lights. Adjusting this allows the smallest, brightest concentration of light to fall on the wound.

Once an operation is underway, it is often necessary to adjust the lights. The surgeon may be working at two different sites, in an operation for varicose veins for instance, turning attention from the groin wound to one further down the leg. It is often difficult to get the lighting just right, especially if you are not very tall and the surgeon is! It is best to get some taller and preferably skilled help from someone who is used to the lights. Failing that, you could stand on a footstool.

If you do move the lights, never do so without the scrub nurse's knowledge, and take great care not to desterilize any equipment. Mind people's heads, too! If there is still not adequate light, most suites also have a portable lamp which can be used. As with all other furniture in the theatre, it is good to practise moving the lights and experimenting with the focus when the theatre is empty.

Anaesthetic scavenging

Most theatres these days have scavenging equipment. You will probably have noticed a long length of corrugated plastic tubing somewhere in the theatre, which is part of this system. During long operations this tubing is connected to the anaesthetic circuit at one end, while the other connects to a vent in the ceiling or wall. The system draws out of the theatre any anaesthetic gases or agents leaking from the circuit and which pollute the atmosphere. A build-up of these substances in the air is thought to affect the health of theatre staff adversely. (See Chapter 13 for more detail on the effects of anaesthetic gases.)

The swab rack

This is a metal piece of furniture used for hanging up swabs during an operation for ease of counting. It comprises several tiers, which are usually removable for easy cleaning and autoclaving. There is a shelf at the bottom and the whole thing is on wheels so that it is easily moved to wherever it can be seen by the scrub nurse. The separate tiers have either hooks on which to hang the swabs, or else holes to poke them through. The hooks and holes are grouped in numbers of fives, and each tier can usually accommodate ten swabs. The tier system allows for different types of swab to be hung separately, so as to avoid confusion when counting.

When you hang swabs, be careful only to hang one at a time. (Once swabs are wet and screwed up it is not always obvious where one ends and another one begins.) If there are tapes on the swabs, these should be hung in such a way as to be clearly visible for counting. The tapes are an extra safety check, since it will have been established that each large swab had a tape attached at the beginning of the operation. The rack can also be used for displaying discarded instruments, and the shelf for used receivers belonging to the scrub nurse's set of instruments.

The swab board

Adjacent to the swab rack you will find a white board with a selection of Chinagraph pencils and washable felt markers. This is for recording the amount of blood loss during the operation. It is not used for every operation, but for major surgery where the blood loss is such that some replacement will be required; and particularly during surgery on babies and small children, where what seems a minimal loss can have considerable effect. The nurses record this information for the anaesthetist's benefit, since it is the anaesthetist who will instigate replacement therapy.

The board is usually marked in two columns; one for blood loss from swabs and one for loss from suction. Occasionally other information may also be recorded. The anaesthetist may ask for a running total of urine output to be kept for some catheterized patients, for instance. Take care to ensure that the information is always largely and clearly written, and that the different running totals do not become confused. Remember that the anaesthetist is usually at the opposite end of the theatre to you and the information is for his or her benefit. The scrub nurse may also ask you to record certain information on the board, such as 'one large swab in the wound'. This acts as an aide-mémoire. (Some hospitals use the swab board for recording all the information relating to the swab and needle counts. If this is so in your case, see Chapters 8 and 9 for an account of the relevant procedures.)

Weighing scales: estimating blood loss

You may be rather surprised to see a friendly looking pair of kitchen scales in the operating theatre. So far we have discussed keeping running totals of blood loss, but nothing has been mentioned about how this is estimated. This is where the kitchen scales come in. Next to the scales you should find a list of the known dry weights of each different type of swab. To estimate blood loss, you weigh the blood-soaked swab, and from that weight subtract the known dry weight. This leaves you with the weight of blood lost, which is the amount you record, adding it to your running total. For example, if a large swab is known to weigh 20 g when dry and when soaked in blood it registers 90 g on the scales, then the extra 70 g must be the weight of blood lost; it cannot be anything else. As 1 g is the weight of 1 ml of water or blood, a blood loss of 70 g therefore indicates that the volume the patient has lost is 70 ml. If a swab does become wet from any other fluid (perhaps water or saline used to wash the wound) the scrub nurse will inform you. This swab will not need to be weighed.

To estimate the blood loss from suction, simply record the amount registered on the side of the suction bottle and add it to your running total. This can be done at say, half-hourly intervals during a long operation, or more frequently if the amount of blood lost is rising rapidly. If the blood in the bottle is mixed with water or saline, the scrub nurse will tell you how much extra fluid has been put into the wound. This amount is then subtracted from that registered on the suction bottle to give the amount of blood lost.

When operating on babies or small children, the kitchen scales may not be adequate for registering the small amounts of blood lost. Your department will probably have a more sensitive set to be used for this purpose.

The scales can also be used for weighing specimens. In

operations such as a reduction mammoplasty, the surgeon may use the scales to ensure an equal reduction on both sides. After transurethral prostatectomy the surgeon may like to gauge the size of the enlarged gland by weighing the pieces of excised tissue – a kind of trophy-hunting instinct!

X-ray screens

Every theatre has an x-ray screen situated by the light control panel. This is vital as some operations are conducted with close reference to a patient's x-rays throughout. This is especially true of emergency orthopaedic surgery, tumour surgery and operations such as cholecystectomy, where a peroperative cholangiogram is performed. (You will certainly appreciate how important it is to ensure that patients' x-rays accompany them when they go down to theatre when you return to ward work.)

Rubbish bins, swab bins and linen skips

Every theatre has separate disposal containers for rubbish, swabs and linen. The swabs are eventually discarded with the rest of the rubbish, but during the operation they must remain separate, to facilitate the swab-counting procedure (see Chapter 9, for a full description of swab-counting). Should any discrepancies arise, it is easier and more hygienic to search through a bag containing only swabs, rather than swabs mixed with a lot of other rubbish. *No swabs should leave the theatre at all during the operation* for this reason. Once a bag of swabs is taken to the sluice room, it is hard to distinguish it from the swabs of the last operation, and the scrub team can never then be absolutely sure that their swab count is accurate. So leave all the disposal bags in the theatre until the end of the operation, and the scrub nurse has told you that he or she is entirely happy with the final count. Then the swab bag can be tied and placed inside the ordinary rubbish bag. Fresh disposal bags are always brought in for every operation.

These are the main pieces of furniture found in every operating theatre, and those which you need to become familiar with.

Before leaving the empty department, let us just have a brief look at the *Recovery* area. Over the past few years there has been increasing recognition of the value of specialized recovery areas. Recovery was once carried out in the corridor outside the operating theatre; now all immediately postoperative patients are brought together to the area known as recovery, where they are nursed by specially trained staff. By the time patients return to the ward, they are out of danger of immediate anaesthetic and surgical complications. There is even a growing trend for recovery areas to offer a 24-hour service, to cater for those patients who would normally be transferred to the intensive therapy unit postoperatively.

Recoveries are normally made up of several bed spaces, each with the necessary equipment to facilitate recovery.

Every space will have a supply of *oxygen*, which is prescribed for virtually every postoperative patient. This ensures that the blood is fully oxygenated, even if breathing is only very shallow. The oxygen supply may be piped through the wall, or it may be used directly from a cylinder. Every supply has a flowmeter, to show the rate in litres per minute at which the oxygen is administered. The usual rate is 4–5 litres. There is a handle on the side of the meter which regulates flow. Disposable tubing and masks, or nasal cannulae if they are more appropriate, are attached just below the flowmeter. These must be changed for each patient.

Suction, which by now you are becoming familiar with, is also vital for every bed space. The patient's airway must be kept clear of mucus in order for the oxygen to have good effect. There is also a tendency for patients to vomit postoperatively as a reaction to the anaesthetic drugs.

More familiar to you will be the *stethoscope and sphygmomanometer* for the regular blood pressure recordings.

The recovery is stocked with much more equipment (discussed in greater detail in Chapter 10). For the time being it is enough to have noticed the above four items which feature most in the recovery of patients – oxygen supply, suction apparatus, stethoscope and sphygmomanometer. There is one other piece of apparatus which should be located immediately however – the *emergency trolley*. Every recovery has a trolley equipped with all that is necessary to deal with cardiac arrests or anaesthetic emergencies. There will be a defibrillator and all the emergency drugs, syringes, needles, intravenous infusion equipment and strappings which are found in the ward emergency boxes. There will also be a laryngoscope, a selection of oral airways and intubation equipment. Most of this is already familiar to you, but do ensure that when you work in recovery, you take a fresh look at the instructions for defibrillator use. Intubation equipment will be fully discussed in Chapter 5. Should an emergency occur in the recovery, or anywhere in the operating department, there are usually plenty of anaesthetists and other medical staff at hand. It is therefore not necessary to instigate the hospital emergency procedure through the central switchboard. There may however be exceptions, perhaps when patients are recovering during unsocial hours or at weekends. Find out the policy for your operating department.

3

Who's who in the operating department

You now have some idea of the nature of the physical environment and how it works. Let us now people the landscape, and look at who makes up this multidisciplinary bustle.

THE NURSING STAFF

We'll start with the most familiar people. The nursing hierarchy in the operating department is the same as on the wards. Each operating list is the responsibility of a sister or charge nurse, usually helped by at least one other trained nurse. The nurses are normally allocated either to one particular theatre or else to specific surgeons' lists. Either way, their work should encompass a variety of surgical experience, with the exception of highly specialized areas like cardiothoracic or neurosurgery. There is usually a core of trained staff on night duty, often supplemented by day staff on call to cover emergencies. Anaesthetic and recovery nurses often have a separate hierarchy and work rota, as the pace of their work and their busy periods tend to differ from those of the nurses working in theatres. The two disciplines together make up the nursing staff of the operating department.

There may also be trained nurses in your department undertaking a National Board course in either operating department nursing, or less frequently, in anaesthetics. The former course lasts 54 weeks, the latter 6 months. These nurses have greater mobility within the department in order for them to gain the fullest variety of experience. Unlike learner nurses, they are not supernumerary students; the department often seems sparsely staffed when they have a study day.

The number of National Board students will of course vary, depending on how many your department can comfortably absorb. Their presence and yours will ensure a range of teaching skills from which you can both benefit: from a course tutor, clinical teacher or perhaps a sister or charge nurse with special teaching responsibilities.

You will have noticed by now that there is a very high concentration of trained nurses working within the operating department. Compared with other areas, it appears 'top-heavy' with sisters and charge nurses. This is purely on paper however; in practice it never seems so. This is indicative of the nature of the work, which incorporates intensive patient care, a high teaching input and considerable management responsibilities.

Another interesting aspect of operating department nursing is that the power balance which exists between nursing and medical staff is different from anything you will have experienced before. Since the Griffiths Report (see Glossary) it is now possible to have a theatre manager without a nursing or medical background, but as yet this is only the case in about two hospitals throughout the country; the rest are all managed by nurses. Most hospitals have a Theatre Users Committee, where surgeons and anaesthetists join the nurses to discuss policy, but ultimately the nurses are in charge. Unlike on the wards, where a nursing officer cannot prevent medical staff from admitting patients to the department, theatre nurses have the power of veto. All operating lists must have their approval. On the question of emergency and out of normal working hours surgery, medical staff may decide in which order this should be done, but the nurses decide on when and where. These decisions are based on what is available to them in terms of staff, equipment and time. Of course they are not made in isolation; good communications and diplomacy are vital when co-operating with medical staff, or these decisions would not be respected. You will find that theatre nurses are very powerful in their own department, which makes for very interesting internal politics!

Operating department assistants (ODAs)

This is a grade of staff which will be new to you. ODAs undertake a 2-year City and Guilds training course in operating department technique: a year of surgical and a year of anaesthetic experience. The grade came into being as part of the recommendations of the Lewen Report (1970), London: HMSO. Throughout the 1960s there had been a chronic shortage of nurses in the operating department, with the result that those in post were very pressurized and lacking in administrative support. The other mainstay of the theatre team at that time were the technicians. They too suffered due to the lack of nursing staff, but they also had more fundamental grievances. They wanted a more detailed and standardized training with suitable financial incentives.

The upshot of this dissatisfactory situation was that a government inquiry was instigated. The committee, which included several nurse representatives, was chaired by Walpole Lewen, an eminent neurosurgeon. Their brief was to examine proposals to improve the lot of the theatre nurse already in post, and to find ways of making it a more attractive career to other nurses.

The committee identified the major problem of theatre nurses as not having enough time to nurse. They lacked the freedom of time to care for patients, as they were constrained by too many non-nursing duties requiring attention within the department. To rectify the situation the committee created the grade of ODA. The 2-year training would mean that ODAs were of a suitable calibre to rank alongside the nursing staff and to be interchangeable with them. The workload which had hitherto been the sole burden of the theatre nurse could effectively be shared. This solution also greatly pleased the technicians. It was decided at this time however, that a nurse should remain in overall charge of the operating department.

Entry requirements for the new grade were evidence of a good general education, but each training school still has its own criteria for selection. A basis for the training programme was also proposed, to include a sound understanding of all aspects of the operating department and hospital organization, and an insight into ethical standards associated with patient care. ODAs were also to gain knowledge of the use and maintenance of a vast range of equipment, including electric, electronic and mechanical apparatus, surgical instruments and other anaesthetic equipment. Most of the 2 years were to be spent within the operating department, but some time was set aside for allocations to the wards and other relevant departments. Nurses were to be very much involved in training ODAs.

Once qualified, ODAs normally opt to remain in either surgery or anaesthetics only; the latter seems to be the most popular choice. After a further 2 years, an ODA with good management and teaching skills can be promoted to the rank of senior operating department assistant (SODA). There is a limited number of these posts however. Each department decides how many it can accommodate; a large department of 10–12 suites may only have 2 or 3 SODAs. Some are absorbed back into ODA training schemes, where a few co-ordinator posts exist around the country.

Initially ODAs were represented by the Ancillary Staffs Council. Since 1984 they have transferred to the Professional and Technical Council – evidence of their growing skill, expertise and established professional status.

MEDICAL STAFF

Anaesthetists

These are the doctors who specialize in giving anaesthetics, caring for the artificially ventilated and resuscitating patients. It is not surprising therefore that most of their time is spent in the operating department. They make few appearances on the wards, except to visit preoperative patients or as part of the 'crash team'. The other place where they do spend a lot of time is the intensive therapy unit. Here, with a high proportion of ventilated patients requiring constant supervision for the maintenance of life, they have evolved as the natural medical managers. Increasingly in the last decade they have also become experts in the field of pain control. Techniques for delivering very accurate and successful local anaesthetics, often under x-ray control, have been developed. This has led to the creation of many pain control clinics throughout the country, offering invaluable help to sufferers of intractable pain, often associated with cancer.

You will meet a range of anaesthetists in the department, from junior house officers to consultants. During the hours of planned surgery, the juniors normally work under more senior guidance. Once competent however, it is often they who will cover emergency out of hours work, with more senior anaesthetists on call. In theory, during daytime operating lists, consultant anaesthetists are allocated to cover consultant surgeons' lists, registrars to cover registrars, and so on.

It is always dangerous to generalize, but traditionally anaesthetists have received a better press than surgeons in terms of temperament. They have been viewed as more down to earth, more able to help themselves, and generally more affable, cheerful and relaxed. Nurses have always found them less formidable, and they are affectionately referred to as the 'gasmen'. Of course one is tempted to ask why this should be. Is the level of stress in their work lower? It is because there is a much higher percentage of women in anaesthetics than surgery? Is it because anaesthesia evolved as a specialty much later than surgery and is therefore much less ridden with hierarchical prejudice? These are all interesting questions, but of course it is dangerous to generalize. There are always exceptions to every rule.

In arranging planned and emergency surgery, the needs and wishes of the anaesthetists frequently concur with those of the nursing staff. They are conscious of the need to stay within prescribed time limits for planned surgery, in order to be able to provide cover for emergencies, and also to enable them to fulfil all their other responsibilities around the hospital. These common needs have meant that anaesthetists have traditionally been powerful allies of the nursing staff.

> In the theatre he was God. Everything in the routine for operating sessions was arranged to suit his convenience. A white linen suit, freshly starched, was carefully warmed by the junior nurse before being laid out in his changing room in the morning. A thermos pitcher of iced water labelled 'Sir Lancelot Spratt only' was set on a silver tray nearby. He had his own masks, his own scrubbing brush and his own soap. When he crossed the theatre floor from the scrub up basins to the table the onlookers scattered before him like unarmed infantry in front of a tank. If anyone got in his way he simply kicked them out of it. He rarely asked for an instrument but expected the sister to guess which one to place in his waiting hand. If she made a mistake, he calmly dropped the wrong instrument onto the floor. Should she do no better at her second attempt he repeated his little trick. Once he silently reduced a whole trayful of instruments to an unsterile heap at his feet, and the Sister had hysterics (Gordon, 1961).

Surgeons

If anaesthetists are the allies, does this imply that surgeons must be the enemy? Thankfully this is not true, although in the past they have often earned themselves a reputation for being unreasonable selfish workaholics who need to be held in check. Looking back through history, it is not suprising that the image they have projected has been so appalling. During the bulk of the past century they wielded supreme power over surgical patients and nursing staff, who would not dare to question their authority. This of course bred arrogance, added to which surgeons also prided themselves on being 'men of action', as opposed to the cautious physicians who in their view sat on the fence. The standard of their work is not in dispute here, but a cavalier attitude is always unacceptable.

In recent years, however, there have been several changes which have naturally curbed some of their power. Nurses and the new grade ODAs form a better trained and educated theatre team, not afraid to question surgical practice. Other branches of medicine have also mushroomed, and taken some of the surgeons' former glory with them. The expanding role of anaesthetists has already been mentioned, and now others, such as radiologists, are increasingly perfecting operative techniques, such as the embolectomy. The general trend over recent years in favour of non-invasive treatment where posssible indicates that the role of the surgeon is bound to continue shrinking.

> For 30 years Sir Lancelot had a say in everything at St Swithin's from the choice of a new consultant to the choice of a new floor polish, until he thought getting his own way there as natural as the law of gravity and just as convenient for the orderly planning of human affairs (Gordon, 1961).

Changes in health service management have had the same effect. There is now multidisciplinary sharing of responsibilities, and the most recent innovation, the introduction of the general manager who does not necessarily have a health service background, indicates irreversible diminution of the surgeons' administrative power. A dramatic growth in consumer power is another modern phenomenon. The general public is now very aware of its rights as a patient and no longer in awe of surgeons. As in the USA, this country is seeing an increase in litigation involving surgeons and anaesthetists – as well as nurses.

So the surgeon of the late 1980s is a far more enlightened, respectful and personable member of the operating team, aware that like everyone else he or she is there to give a service, to do a specific job. It is rare now to find a surgeon throwing tantrums or instruments at junior staff. The archetypal Sir Lancelot Spratt no longer exists, but perhaps his ghost still lingers.

> Every Tuesday and Thursday afternoon he operated in his own theatre on the top floor. The list for the session was pinned up outside like a music-hall bill – the best cases were always at the top for Sir Lancelot to operate on himself, and the programme degenerated into a string of such minor surgical chores as the repair of hernias and the removal of varicose veins, to be done by his assistants when he

had gone off to his club for a glass of sherry before dinner (Gordon, 1961).

The surgeons are organized in firms, as are all other medical staff. Operating lists are arranged in the name of the consultant who should appear to operate or to oversee the juniors operating. Records are kept in the department of the preferences of each surgeon, with regard to equipment and procedures, which are met as far as possible. House officers also come to theatre to assist with surgery. It should be remembered that they often need supervision in basic theatre behaviour, i.e. scrubbing and gowning, maintaining a sterile field and aseptic technique.

There are still some areas of tension which exists between surgeons and nursing staff. Time-keeping, already referred to, is a sore point. Over-stepping prescribed time limits for surgery results in an over-stretched, over-stressed nursing staff, which can have dangerous repercussions. Increasingly records of this are being kept which, with the aid of computers, can be stored and analysed over a period of time to see just how big a problem this is. This will no doubt bring about beneficial change. Communications are also a persistent problem. There is still much room for improvement on the part of surgeons in understanding that nurses need prior warning if they are to provide specialized equipment or care.

Lingering attitudes of the past still cause problems. Conservatism can be difficult, especially in teaching hospitals. A surgeon who only likes to work with familiar staff and who does not welcome a new face severely limits the opportunities for new staff to learn. Despite the many changes in recent years, surgeons are still predominantly men. Obstetrics and gynaecology has attracted a few women surgeons, but in other fields women are not well represented. Nurses, too, are still predominantly women, so sexist tension and male chauvinism remain the problems they always were.

This does all sound rather like a battlefield, and in many ways it has been. Theatre nurses have come a long way in their fight for respect and fair consideration, but the areas outlined above show that the fight is not yet over. The ultimate aim is for good teamwork, which operates through mutual respect and good communication. The benefits of this are enormous: good patient care, an enjoyable and satisfying work atmosphere and the elimination of unnecessary stress.

Domestic staff

Their role in the department is very important as high standards of cleanliness are vital. They are specially trained to work here by their supervisors, who maintain close links with the nursing officers for infection control. They therefore have a good understanding of the concept of cross-infection and are knowledgeable about which detergents and disinfectants are appropriate for which cleaning jobs.

During the hours of routine surgery, the domestics keep the areas outside the suites and the sluice rooms clear, while the theatre itself, the anaesthetic room and the clean preparation room are usually the responsibility of the nursing staff. At night all the operating suites are thoroughly cleaned by the domestic staff.

Some hospitals employ *operating department orderlies*, (ODOs) who perform a wider range of duties. They are more highly trained, and will clean the operating theatres between cases, removing soiled linen and rubbish, as well as performing the other domestic staff duties. They also receive training in lifting and positioning patients for surgery and for working in the theatre sterile supplies unit (TSSU) where they clean, pack, autoclave and maintain instruments.

Porters

Theatre porters form a very important link between the isolated operating department and the rest of the hospital. Their duties are very varied, including collecting and returning patients to and from the wards, as well as lifting, positioning and turning them on their sides. They will move heavy machinery and perform numerous errands to the pharmacy, pathology department and blood transfusion in particular. They may also have some cleaning duties. A reliable and experienced theatre porter is a very valuable commodity.

Receptionists

Most large departments now employ at least one receptionist to perform clerical and secretarial work. As intermediaries between theatre staff and those wishing to make contact from outside, either by telephone or in person, they too are invaluable. They are usually responsible for the ordering and distribution of stationery and the long-term maintenance of theatre records. With the ever-increasing workload in the operating theatre, the need for clerical back-up has grown considerably. In fact the job of theatre receptionist or secretary could be infinitely expanded to include all kinds of other responsibilities, such as overseeing catering arrangements, laundry supplies, other types of ordering and booking emergency cases. The limits of the job reflect the needs of the department and the calibre and interest of the person in the post. At best, receptionists form the nerve centre of theatre operations.

Radiographers

These are frequent visitors to the operating department, as it is often necessary to take x-rays during the course of surgery to gauge a surgeon's progress. They have received instructions about asepsis and maintaining the sterile field, as the nature of their work brings them into close contact with it. Most departments are equipped with all the apparatus for taking and developing x-rays.

Photographers

They come to the operating theatre to take photographs, or increasingly videos, of interesting specimens or new procedures for the department of medical illustration. Their work also requires them to come into close proximity with the wound and sterile field, and hence they often need reminding of the principles of asepsis.

Technicians

A host of technicians of all kinds come to the operating department. Some are not hospital staff, but are employed by private companies to carry out periodic maintenance on specific pieces of equipment, such as anaesthetic machines and operating microscopes. A hospital electrician will make regular visits to check operating lights and other appliances. Plumbers, locksmiths, carpenters and engineers who service the autoclaves will also appear from time to time, as in other departments.

Other visitors

The operating department has a constant stream of other visitors, not accounted for above. Students of all disciplines come to watch surgery. Medical representatives come to demonstrate new equipment, in the hope of making sales. Midwives and paediatricians come to attend births by caesarean section. Medical and nursing staff from other hospitals or countries come to learn about different techniques. With such a mixture of people coming and going, it is not surprising that you feel confused at first. One thing to remember about such visitors is that they all need some supervision about how to dress and how to behave in the operating department.

But how do you tell who is who?

This is a familiar cry of the new student nurse. Try to establish as soon as possible the ways in which your hospital distinguishes the different grades of staff. Different coloured disposable hats are commonly used, and are effective in distinguishing different grades of nurses, ODAs and trainees. Some hospitals use coloured belts in this manner. When it comes to medical staff it is usually much harder to tell who is who. They tend to resist such attempts at identification, preferring to remain anonymous. Still, initially the medical staff are of secondary importance for you; their names and grades will become familiar in time.

The importance of name badges cannot be over-estimated. They leave you in no doubt as to exactly who you are dealing with, and what their role is. Remember always to wear yours. Some hospitals also have a system of coloured spots for students to wear on their name badges, which indicate the number of weeks they have worked in the department. This gives the trained staff some idea of what can be expected of their students. If this would make you feel more secure, why not suggest it is introduced in your hospital?

The trained staff, even if you do not know them initially, will have a much better idea of who you are. However, even if you are wearing a name badge, don't leave that to do all the work for you. It is only polite to introduce yourself to new colleagues, and while you are doing this, explain how long you will be working with them and what stage you are at in your basic training. This will make far more of an impression on busy theatre staff, who appreciate a more assertive student. Do this whenever you are working with new colleagues, and they will soon remember who you are.

Identity is important to make you feel less alienated in this new department, but it is also important for security reasons. The theatres house a lot of very expensive equipment, which may tempt thieves. If you see anyone acting suspiciously or an unfamiliar face, do not be afraid to confront them and ask them what they are doing, or ask a senior member of staff to do so. If they are a member of hospital staff or working for a legitimate contractor they should be able to furnish you with adequate identification. If not, speak to the nurse in charge who should alert the hospital security officer.

Enjoy this rare chance to be a member of such a multi-disciplinary family of staff. You will find teamwork can be very satisfying and a lot of fun. You will gain in confidence through working amongst different disciplines, and also through having contact with some very senior hospital staff. Take the opportunity to learn from these people. Observe how they apply theory in the practical situation; observe their management and interpersonal skills. You will also gain an interesting insight into hospital politics!

References

Gordon, R. (1961). *Doctor in the House*, Harmondsworth: Penguin Books, pp. 58, 64, 71.

Further reading

Darbyshire, P. (1987). The burden of history. *Nursing Times/Nursing Mirror*, **83**, 4, January 28, pp. 28–37.

Dimond, B. (1987). Your disobedient servant, nurses and doctors. *Nursing Times/Nursing Mirror*, **83**, 4, January 28, pp. 28–37.

Smoyak, S. (1987). Redefining roles. *Nursing Times/Nursing Mirror*, **83**, 4, January 28, pp. 28–37.

4

How to behave in the operating department

The aim of this chapter is not to be patronizing, but to help those of you who are new to the department and afraid of doing the wrong thing. This is a very understandable fear, as there is nothing much familiar about this place. It has the air of being governed by many strict and yet invisible rules. You feel loath to take the initiative, as criteria upon which you would normally base your judgements perhaps do not apply here. In an effort to redress some of this uncertainty, let us take a look at a few areas where certain rules can be identified.

DRESS

One thing you will become more acutely aware of during your operating department allocation is that your own body is a very potent contaminator and source of infection. The aims of theatre clothing are twofold. One is to render your body less likely to contaminate the clean department and sterile operating fields. The second is to prevent sparks of static electricity emanating from clothing or footwear, which could lead to explosions.

Light, usually cotton, dresses or trousers and tops are provided for you to wear, and there will be storage space for your outdoor clothing. Trousers and tops have gained in popularity recently, as there is a belief that female staff shed a lot of organisms from the perineum. Therefore trousers with close fitting cuffs around the ankle are especially effective for sealing in these potential contaminants. If dresses are provided, you will probably be required to wear tights, which are considered to be effective for this purpose also. If you wear trousers and tops, be sure to see that the top is securely tucked in. A flapping, loose top is more likely to desterilize surfaces. You should feel comfortable in these outfits, and the many attractive colours and designs now available allow you to take pride in your appearance.

Footwear will also be provided – sandals, clogs or canvas shoes. Their common salient feature is that their soles are made of an anti-static material.

As part of your new self-awareness, you will come to realize that your head and hair, like the perineum, are another major source of shed organisms and dead tissue. For this reason, your hair must be completely covered before you enter the operating department. Disposable paper *hats* are commonly in use now, which are cool, comfortable and brightly coloured. (If your hospital differentiates grades of staff by hat colour, be sure to select the right one, or you could be making difficulties for yourself!)

Finally, before you enter a clean corridor, always wash your hands. You will have been handling your outdoor clothing and your hair, and you are now going to be handling sterile packets. Check that you are wearing your name badge in a prominent position, and that you have a pen. A pen is vital as you will be filling in patient records and labelling specimens. Scissors are also useful for cutting strapping, and a fob watch is a good idea if you are going to be working in anaesthetics or recovery. Theatre clothing is still part of hospital uniform, and you should not be wearing any jewellery except a wedding ring. This is for the same reasons that apply in other departments: jewellery can injure patients and it may also harbour bacteria. If you are going to scrub up, you will need to remove your ring, so make sure that you have a strong safety pin with which to fasten it inside your pocket.

Before you enter an operating suite where sterile packs are open, you must put on a *face mask*. Your nose and mouth are another potent source of infection. Masks act as a filter. Disposable ones are most commonly in use, but cotton ones are available if you find that you have an allergic reaction to them. They should be handled by the fastening tapes only, as once used, the material of the mask is saturated with the vapour of your breath and any exhaled organisms. They should be changed every time you leave and then re-enter a suite, and not worn dangling round your neck. They should be disposed of in the bags for infected rubbish. Masks are only effective for a period of about 2 hours, after which time they will be saturated and unable to filter air.

The combination of wearing hats and masks has the drawback of muffling sounds and speech. You may find that it is often difficult to hear instructions, which is doubly difficult when the terminology is also unfamiliar. Never be afraid to ask for things to be repeated. Conversely, you must remember to speak up for yourself a little louder than normal, and enunciate clearly.

HEALTH MATTERS

If you are suffering from an infection or have an infected lesion you should not be on duty in the operating department; you are too much of a hazard to surgical patients. If you have any doubts about this, the best thing to do is to telephone your nursing officer and ask for advice. It may be that you could be safely allocated to work elsewhere as a temporary measure.

Smoking is obviously a dangerous habit in the operating department. It has already been mentioned that there are large quantities of inflammable substances stored here and there is a heavy emphasis upon the need for fire prevention. Separate rest rooms for smokers are usually provided, and you should restrict your habit to this area only.

NOISE

Noise in the operating department is a great stressor for both patients and staff. It jars on fragile nerves and breaks concentration. The golden rule here is to be as quiet as possible at all times. Consideration of the anxiety felt by conscious patients in the department must be paramount in governing your behaviour. When a patient is awake in the anaesthetic room or theatre, aside from quiet reassurance from a nurse, there should be the absolute minimum of noise from equipment and staff. Equally, when patients are being induced into a state of anaesthesia, remember that the hearing is always the last sense to go, and the first to reappear. Patients should always be addressed with the utmost respect and you should carefully consider what you say in their presence. Confidential information regarding their condition and prognosis should certainly not be discussed over them. Remember this also when you come to work in recovery, and are giving the ward nurse a 'hand-over'.

Surgeons, anaesthetists and scrub nurses also need careful consideration. During a long operation, when there is not much for the circulating assistants to do, the temptation is always to chat. This is not helped by the large volume of visitors the department gets, which render it a rather sociable place. You will no doubt be faced with this dilemma.

Quiet conversation is normally permissible, provided it is not distracting. It must also not impair your awareness of the progress of the operation or your ability to respond to the needs of your colleagues. You must become sensitive to the different stages of an operation. Exposure of a wound is normally fairly routine, but once the site of operation is exposed, greater concentration is needed to carry out the necessary procedure. Once this is completed and the wound is being closed, the atmosphere again lightens, for this too is normally fairly routine. Unexpected difficulties can arise at any time however, be they surgical or anaesthetic, and at these times you should keep absolute silence until the crisis is over. You must be ready to hear and act quickly upon any instructions. Until you become attuned to the different moods of surgery, be guided by the scrub nurse. He or she can let you know when it is suitable to talk quietly or ask questions, and when it is not.

You may be rather surprised to discover that some theatres play music during surgery. Usually it is classical and played quietly, and of course only if the surgeon allows it. The soothing effects of the music have to be carefully weighed in the balance against the fact that a form of noise has been introduced to the theatre.

You will be even more surprised to discover that sometimes the atmosphere in a theatre can be very noisy, even raucous. This does occasionally happen when a theatre has a list of very minor, routine surgery, and the surgeon is particularly happy; usually on a Friday afternoon! In such an atmosphere it is of course suitable to respond, taking your cue from the surgeon, but never be the unsolicited initiator of a lot of noise.

By all means enjoy your time in the operating department, responding to those around you and sharing in a relaxed, happy atmosphere. Do however be sensitive to changes of mood, and do learn to regulate the amount of noise you make accordingly. Recognize that unnecessary noise does cause stress, and not just talking. Banging doors, ringing telephones and moving equipment can all be very distracting. At times the atmosphere in a theatre can be so intense that even the rustling of a paper bag can be too much. As you become more sensitive you will become more proficient in other means of communication – learning to give sign language with your eyes and hands, with eloquent effect.

MAINTAINING A STERILE FIELD

Once you are inside the operating suite, correctly dressed and having entered via the clean preparation room, you must learn to take extra care to avoid desterilizing equipment. Once something is no longer sterile it cannot be used, as the risk of introducing wound infection is too great. Desterilizing equipment means loss of time and greater expense as replacements must be found. This is not always easy, especially where rare equipment is concerned. It may be that the whole scrub team has to wait for instruments to be put through the autoclave again. Meanwhile the patient is receiving a much longer anaesthetic than is necessary, and the whole operating list is running late. The scrub nurse is put under added stress, as he or she must begin to lay up the trolley all over again, and the general atmosphere is one of frustration. So desterilizing equipment is something to be avoided as far as possible.

The rule is that normally anything green is sterile, and should not be touched. This includes drapes on trolleys and patients, and the green gowns worn by the scrub team. The other golden rule is that if you are not sure, don't touch; ask first. Having established which things are sterile, you must then imagine an invisible barrier 45–60 cm deep around each trolley or person. You must not move within this barrier, or sterile aura if you like, as it is then that you are at risk of desterilizing the objects. Modify your movements in the clean preparation room and the theatre accordingly, and give anything green a wide berth.

At the beginning of an operation, when trolleys and personnel are more mobile, extra care must be taken. If you are helping the scrub nurse to wheel the trolleys into position, grip them on bare metal 45–60 cm from the sterile surface. Remember the invisible barrier! Really, you need to develop eyes in the back of the head. Be careful not to move impulsively, and never step backwards without looking to see that there is nothing sterile behind you first. At all times you need to be keenly aware of the position of all sterile surfaces in the theatre.

The hands of the scrub team must be the cleanest part of them, since it is the hands which will be working inside the patient's wound. Take special care therefore if a scrubbed person hands you anything to be removed from the sterile field. To minimize the risk of desterilization, take hold of that object at the point furthest away from their gloved hands.

When opening sterile packages for the scrub nurse, stand well back beyond the invisible barrier, and let him or her take the objects from you using forceps. One thing you must never do is to come between the scrub nurse and trolley; you risk desterilizing both of them.

Visualize the invisible barrier when you are moving equipment too. Don't push the diathermy machine in too closely to the scrub nurse's trolley, and watch that you don't desterilize anything when you move lights or stand on a stool to watch the operation. (Check again that your top is securely tucked into your trousers!) Be careful when diathermy or light leads are handed out to you for connection. Do not touch the sterile drapes and mind the scrub nurse's hands. Take hold of the leads at their very opposite ends.

Other things at risk of being desterilized are autoclaves or soaking trays in the clean preparation room. Do not touch these unless you have been told that they are no longer needed for the rest of the operating list.

Finally, never touch the scrub nurse's trolley at the end of an operation until he or she tells you that you may. Unforeseen events sometimes occur. It may become evident that there is still bleeding inside a wound, which will necessitate re-opening. If this happens, the scrub nurse will need all the instruments again. Wait until you are told that sterile equipment is finished with and can be touched.

There is much to consider in maintaining a sterile field. You will need to concentrate and be vigilant at all times. Should you accidentally desterilize anything, or see someone else do so, you must always say. The preceding observations may put you off, but remember that you are still the patient's advocate. Their health and well-being must always take priority over saving your own skin. It helps to imagine that every patient could be someone close to you; your mother, father, sister, boyfriend. Once you start to think like this, you will not remain silent for long. No patient should suffer a wound infection unnecessarily, and it would be shameful if they did because you were afraid to speak out. Yes, it takes time and money to replace desterilized equipment, but if finance is a major consideration, then it is cheaper to get a fresh set of drapes and instruments immediately than it is to keep a patient in hospital for an extra week with a wound infection. Other staff may show frustration at first, but they will always respect you for saying that you have desterilized something or seen someone else do so. Remember also that anyone can make mistakes. You will obviously need to supervise other students and visitors in the theatre, but sometimes it is senior nurses or senior surgeons who unwittingly contaminate things. Their mistakes should be pointed out just the same, regardless of rank. There is no place for pride when patients have put their trust into your hands.

These are just some guidelines about sterility. Chapter 9 deals more fully with the subject.

The aim of this chapter has been to point out some aspects of good behaviour in the operating department. Knowing a few basic ground rules should save you from that awful feeling of uncertainty and embarrassment – and sometimes trouble.

Further reading

McCluske F. (1983). Music in the operating suite. *NAT News*, **20** (9), pp. 33–40.
Nicholson-Pegg A. (1982). The wearing of wedding rings in the operating department. *NAT News*, **19** (4), pp. 19–25.

5

Anaesthetics

Most learner nurses find working in the anaesthetic room less
alien than other aspects of theatre nursing. Patients are awake
on arrival and really appreciate finding a nurse there to care for
them. So it is here, in this more familiar and comfortable
environment, that a role for the learner nurse in the department
is outlined first.

PREPARATION OF THE ANAESTHETIC ROOM

Before a patient arrives to be anaesthetized, there is a lot of
behind-the-scenes work to be done. Safety checks have to be
carried out on all the equipment to be used, which must be
standing ready in case of emergency and to avoid wasting time.

When you first arrive in the anaesthetic room, you will probably
find that you have been allocated to work with either a trained
nurse or an ODA. Introduce yourself to them, and get them to
show you around, in particular pointing out the most vital pieces
of equipment – suction, intubation equipment and the nearest
defribillator. Then get them to show you how to prepare for an
operating list.

The *anaesthetic machine*, or Boyle's machine, needs attention.
There must be adequate gas in the cylinders, which must be
open, and the oxygen pressure failure alarm must be tested. If
there are piped gases, these must be correctly connected to the
machine. The vaporizers must be checked to ensure that they
contain enough volatile agent, and may need to be refilled. If
you have a machine in the theatre in addition to the one in the
anaesthetic room, then all this needs to be done twice.

You must always check the *suction*, to see that it is working
efficiently, and that clean tubing and a Yankaur suction head
have been affixed. (See Chapter 2 for how to check the suction
equipment.)

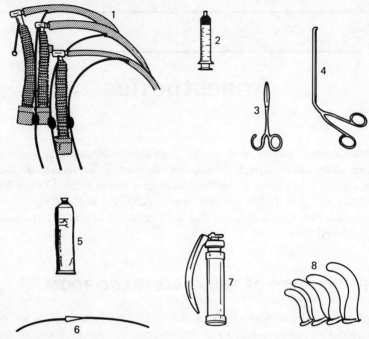

Fig. 5.1 Intubation equipment. **1** Selection of Magill endotracheal tubes with Cobb's connections and catheter mounts. **2** 1 × 10 ml syringe. **3** 1 × 12 cm (5 in) Spencer Wells forceps. **4** Magill forceps. **5** Lubricant jelly. **6** Endotracheal tube introducing stilette. **7** Laryngoscope. **8** Airways

The *intubation tray* must be checked (Fig. 5.1). The laryngoscope must have a clean blade and its light bulb must be working. Local anaesthetic spray for the vocal cords must be available. There should be a selection of appropriate sized endotracheal tubes available (usually a size 8 for a woman, and size 9 for a man. Everyone varies slightly however, so several different sizes need to be put out ready). The endotracheal tubes must be tested for safe functioning, in particular the inflatable cuffs. This is done by injecting a syringeful of air via the pilot tube. Keep the cuff inflated for a few seconds to ensure that there are no leaks; if there are, the tube should be discarded immediately.

Every tube must have an appropriate sized connection fitted into the end. Again, check that these fit snugly, without leaks. Then you must check that the available catheter mount will fit on to these connections. These are the main safety checks; and remember that primarily, you are checking to see that the circuit fits easily but securely together, and that there are no leaks.

Check also that an introducer for the endotracheal tubes is present, and a pair of Magill intubation forceps to remove foreign bodies from the airway. There should be a syringe to inflate the tube cuffs, an artery forceps, with a good grip, to occlude the pilot tube, and some KY or Xylocaine jelly. The intubation procedure is described later in this chapter.

Intubation equipment must always be at hand, even if the surgery to be done is minor and would not normally indicate the need for it. You can never be sure when anaesthetic difficulties will arise, and being able to intubate a patient quickly ensures absolute safety and complete control of breathing.

Alongside the intubation tray you will need to put out a selection of black, anti-static *rubber face masks* for use in induction. These fit on to the end of the black anaesthetic tubing from the machine with the aid of an appropriate sized angled connection. Mount the connections ready on to each mask so they can be used straight away. (Normally a size 4 mask will fit a woman and a size 5 a man; but again, everyone is different, so have a selection available.) You will also need a selection of *oral airways*, usually the Magill or Guedel types (size 2 for a woman and 3 for a man). Nasopharyngeal airways are also commonly used now. These have the advantage of avoiding accidental damage to any crowned teeth. If your anaesthetist likes to use them, the selection you have available should take into account that the normal size for a woman is a 7, and that for a man is 8. The airways must be lubricated for use, so have some KY jelly and anaesthetic green gauze swabs at hand. You should also locate the black rubber *harnesses*, Clausen harnesses, which can be used to retain the face masks.

Syringes, needles and *drug labels* must be available for the anaesthetist, and some of the *drugs* themselves can be collected in readiness, provided of course that they are not controlled drugs. (A list of the preferred drugs for each anaesthetist is normally kept in each anaesthetic room.) The anaesthetist must draw them up ready for use, or else must be present supervising while you or the other assistant do so.

Some kind of *intravenous access* will be necessary, usually a butterfly needle, to start off the anaesthetic. Have this out ready along with a selection of cut lengths of strapping. If the operation indicates the need for an *intravenous infusion*, this can be run through in readiness. Remember always to label infusions with the date and time of preparation, in case they are not used immediately.

Monitoring equipment must be at hand; usually electrodes to record an ECG tracing and a blood pressure cuff and sphygmomanometer. It is also a good idea to collect any pieces of *table equipment* that may be necessary, such as an arm board or lithotomy poles, to save time later on.

There is much to think about and do before the patient arrives, as you can see, and it is all necessary to make anaesthetic administration run smoothly and safely. Of course you will not be expected to know all of this immediately, but gradually you will learn what needs to be done. Then you can set to work before the operating list to check the suction, for example, without having to be supervised or asked.

When the patient does arrive all the preparation should be finished, so that there is an atmosphere of quiet and calm. Most patients will have been premedicated, so they should be disturbed as little as possible. Remember to shut doors to keep out noises and draughts; patients will feel more relaxed if they are warm enough. It is particularly important to remember to shut the doors leading to the theatre. Think of the effect on the poor patient, being confronted by the sight of the theatre still in disarray from the last operation!

RECEIVING PATIENTS

Receiving patients from the ward nurse is a duty which most learners enjoy. It is an extremely important duty, as vital information regarding the patient is passed on. Before you receive your first patient, you need to find out the correct hospital procedure. Have one of the trained staff show you how this works in practice, and then practise under supervision before going it alone. Your hospital procedure should include all of the following points.

Your first duty is to reassure the patients. Remember to take off your face mask before greeting them, so that they can see a friendly, caring face: the face of another nurse. Then you must check the *identity of the patient*, to ensure that you have the right person for the correct operation. The patient's name and registration number are checked on the notes, the patient's wristband and on the operating list. As an extra safety check you can also ask patients what their name is, provided they are awake and able to answer you.

Then you must check the *consent form*. This is a very important legal document: a contract between the patient and the medical staff, giving permission for the operation to take place. Like all legal documents it must be worded in such a way as to be detailed, yet unambiguous and accurate. The name of the operation must be written in full with no abbreviations, and if any additional procedures are deemed likely, they too must be written out in full. For example, if a woman is having a breast lump biopsy which is to be sent for immediate histological examination, on the understanding that if the biopsy contains malignant tissue then a mastectomy will be performed, all of this must be clearly stated on the consent form. The wording of the consent form does also provide for emergencies however. It contains the sentence: 'I also consent to such further or alternative operative measures as may be found to be necessary during the course of the operation and to the administration of a general, local or other anaesthetic for any of these purposes'. Patients do have the right to delete this sentence however, or to add a clause of their own.

The form must be signed by the patient, or the patient's relative or guardian, signifying that they have been given a full explanation of what the operation entails, and also signed by the doctor who has given this explanation. Check that both signatures are present, and that the name of the operation coincides exactly with what is written on the operating list. Pay special attention where either 'right' or 'left' side is stated. Often this can be further verified by checking skin markings at the proposed site of operation. When you have a moment, take the consent form to show the scrub nurse. Together with the surgeon, the scrub nurse is the one who shares the legal liability for the performance of a wrong operation. Any discrepancies regarding the identity of the patient or the consent form should be immediately reported to the nurse in charge.

You must check that the patient has been *nil by mouth* for at least 4 hours, by asking the patient directly, where possible, when he or she last ate or drank. Check that any false teeth or other *prostheses* have been removed, with the exception of hearing aids. These can remain in place until the patient is anaesthetized, so that full reassurance and explanations of what is happening can be given, instead of a very frightening silence. (All items of patients' property removed by you in the anaesthetic room must be carefully stored to avoid being lost.) You must also make a note of any *capped or crowned teeth*. There are two reasons why the anaesthetist needs to know about these. Firstly, he or she will have to take care not to damage them when inserting the laryngoscope, and secondly, should they become detached, they could be inhaled by the patient, with serious consequences.

The *prescription sheet* should be checked to see whether or not the patient was premedicated, and at what time. Any *drug allergies* should be recorded here too. You also need to know if the patient is allergic to any kinds of dressing material or antiseptic lotions which could be used in the theatre.

If the nursing process is being used in your department, you will have had prior warning of any *special nursing requirements* for each patient. If it is not, you must make a quick *assessment* of their general condition, with the help of the ward nurse. You must look at their skin. Do they have pressure sores, or are they thin, elderly or dehydrated and likely to develop them? If so, extra-careful positioning and padding will be necessary on the operating table. Are they obese? If so, they may be difficult to lift, so extra male staff will need to be on hand. Do they have any limb deformities or limited range of movement? Have they recently had joint replacement surgery, so that more care than usual must be taken when handling and positioning their limbs? Are there any appliances in situ, such as intravenous infusions, urinary catheters or colostomy bags? If so, extra stands will be needed in the theatre on which to place them, and a disposal bag and gloves must be available to receive the colostomy bag and its contents. The scrub nurse may also not need to lay up that extra catheterization trolley. Has all jewellery been removed, except a wedding ring? This should also be covered with Micropore tape to prevent its being lost.

Much vital information is established by the nurse who receives a patient from the ward. Any special requirements for care, and again any discrepancies, should be reported immediately to the nurse in charge or the anaesthetist, as appropriate. Good, thorough checking ensures greater safety for each patient. Finally, before the ward nurse leaves, make sure that *x-rays* and any other relevant *investigation reports* are present. The ward nurse should also fill in the patient's details in the *theatre register*. Once the anaesthetist is happy, the ward nurse may leave.

ANAESTHETIC DRUGS

First of all, what exactly is anaesthesia? *The Concise Oxford Dictionary* (5th ed., 1964, OUP) defines it as: 'insensibility to touch or pain. Loss of sensation in a part or in the whole of the body, induced by drugs'. If you asked an anaesthetist what it meant, the answer would probably include one further element – muscle relaxation. Thus the aims of anaesthesia are threefold.

There are three distinct stages in an anaesthetic. Firstly there is the stage of induction, where the patient is induced into a state of light sleep, analgesia and muscle relaxation, if this is required. The second stage is maintenance. This is when the anaesthetic is deepened to ensure that the patient remains pain-free, relaxed and completely unaware throughout surgery. The last step is reversal. As surgery nears completion, drugs are given to help the patient wake up and recover the ability to regain spontaneous and adequate breathing.

Induction agents

These are the drugs given first of all which bring about the state of anaesthesia – light sleep, analgesia and muscle relaxation – if required.

The two drugs most commonly used to induce *light sleep* are the barbiturates methohexitone (Brietal) and thiopentone (Intraval). Non-barbiturates include propanadid (Epontal), ketamine hydrochloride (Ketalar) and propofol (Diprivan.) All of these drugs are given intravenously and are short-acting. The dosage given is worked out in proportion to the weight of the patient.

Analgesia is commonly achieved by the use of intravenous pethidine, phenoperidine (Operidine), Omnopon and fentanyl (Sublimaze). The dosage given depends upon the nature and expected duration of the operative procedure.

Muscle relaxation can either be long- or short-acting. A short-acting drug is suxamethonium (Scoline), which is used to facilitate intubation. Longer-acting muscle relaxants are pancuronium bromide (Pavulon), atracurium (Tracrium), Alloferin, gallamine (Flaxedil) and curare (Tubocurarine). These are used after the patient has been intubated, to allow the patient to be artificially ventilated. All of these drugs are given intravenously. (Curare has an interesting history. It was discovered by South American

Indians who dipped their spears and arrows in it, and thus paralysed and killed their prey!)

Anaesthesia can also be induced by inhalation, using a mixture of the anaesthetic gases and a volatile agent. This is commonly done for the very sick or frail elderly or for children. Normally however, these are used for deepening the anaesthetic.

Anaesthetic gases

The two most commonly used gases are oxygen and nitrous oxide. Nitrous oxide is a weak anaesthetic agent but it has good hypnotic, relaxant and analgesic properties. You will probably have also noticed cylinders of carbon dioxide on the anaesthetic machine. Carbon dioxide is seldom used; its purpose is to stimulate respiration.

Before we go any further, there are a few things you should know about the *cylinders*. They are all distinctly coloured to prevent confusion. The colours are those dictated by the British Standard. Nitrous oxide cylinders are blue, oxygen cylinders are black with a white band around the top and carbon dioxide cylinders are grey. One other commonly found cylinder in the operating department is compressed air, used to operate orthopaedic and dental drills. This cylinder is grey, with a band around the top which is half white and half black.

Another safety feature of the cylinders is the *pin-index system*. At the point where the cylinders attach on to the anaesthetic machine, there are a number of metal pins. These fit into corresponding holes in the valve at the top of the cylinders. Each type of gas has a different pin-index, i.e. a different configuration of pins, so it is impossible to fit any gas cylinder on to an outlet other than its own. This means that past tragedies, where carbon dioxide has been administered in the place of oxygen, for instance, cannot be repeated. Have the ODA or anaesthetic nurse show you how the pin-index system works next time a cylinder is changed.

Volatile agents

These are substances which vaporize readily at room temperature. They are mixed with the gases to deepen and maintain anaesthesia. The most commonly used agents are halothane (Fluothane), Ethrane and isoflurane. These are the drugs most frequently used to anaesthetize patients. This list is not exhaustive however, and you may come across others.

Reversal agents

These are the drugs given to assist the patient in recovering consciousness and adequate spontaneous breathing. They work in two ways. Neostigmine (Prostigmin) is one of the most commonly used agents; it is an antidote to the long-acting muscle relaxants and frees the respiratory muscles from paralysis. Its use must be preceded by atropine however, as it has side-effects of bradycardia and increased production of secretions.

Other common agents, such as naloxone (Narcan) and doxapram (Dopram) work by directly stimulating the respiratory centre in the brain. Narcan also specifically counteracts the effect of the opiate group of drugs. Its use enables the patient to wake up rapidly, but in so doing it may interfere with postoperative analgesia. All of these drugs are given intravenously towards the end of the operation.

This account has concentrated on the broad objectives and different stages of anaesthesia, rather than going into detail about the individual properties of each drug. This has been deliberate, since initially it is more important for you to understand the former. You can learn detail in the clinical setting, by asking the anaesthetist, anaesthetic nurses and ODAs, and by reading the literature supplied with each drug.

INDUCTION OF ANAESTHESIA

It is now your role to reassure and comfort patients throughout the induction of anaesthesia. It helps if you can explain the initial steps of the procedure. Tell patients that an intravenous needle will be inserted, usually into the back of the hand, and that through this will be injected the drugs to send them off to sleep. Patients often like to know details, and especially limits of time. 'How long will it be before I go to sleep? When will I wake up?' and 'Is the anaesthetic painful?' are common questions. You can reassure them on all of these counts.

A lot of hospitals transfer patients on to the operating table once they are asleep, but in this description we will assume that the patient is being anaesthetized on the operating table. Thus the patient can be positioned in the anaesthetic room, so that surgery may commence immediately the table is wheeled into the theatre. Make sure that your patient is comfortable and warm on the operating table. Arm supports are sometimes restful.

The first step in inducing anaesthesia is for the anaesthetist to establish venous access. Usually a butterfly needle is inserted into a vein on the back of the hand. You can assist in this procedure by rendering the patient's veins more prominent and accessible. Squeeze gently above the patient's wrist, temporarily cutting off the venous return from the hand. This has the effect of engorging the veins and making them stand out as an easier target for the anaesthetist's needle. You can also show the patient how to open and close the hand repeatedly like a fist, which speeds up the process.

The next step is for the anaesthetist to check that the needle really is in a vein. You can hand him or her a syringe and needle for this purpose, with which fluid can be withdrawn via the butterfly needle. If blood is withdrawn, the needle is certainly in a vein.

The anaesthetist then needs to secure access. The veins here are small and it is easy for the slightest movement to dislodge the needle, causing its point to puncture the vein wall. So have a piece of cut strapping ready in your hand to pass to the anaesthetist, so that he or she can remain as still as possible until the butterfly needle is secured. You can help set up an intravenous infusion in the same manner.

Once the anaesthetist has verified that the cannula is correctly positioned in the vein, you then need to hand over the end of the infusion tubing, having first removed its protective covering. Once this is connected to the cannula, open the flow control and see that the infusion is running. More strapping is needed here: a narrow piece to secure the juncture of the cannula and vein, and then wider pieces of Elastoplast to splint the tubing to the patient's arm.

Always observe the patient. If he or she feels much pain, the chances are that the cannula is in the tissues, not a vein. Have a supply of green gauze swabs and strapping ready to apply pressure over points from which tissued cannulae have to be removed.

Once access is established, the anaesthetist will inject the induction agents. You can be ready to hand over the different syringes the anaesthetist has prepared, removing the needles as necessary. Remember to be very quiet now. Even though the patient will soon be lightly asleep, hearing is always the last sense to go. As always, observe the patient. When he or she begins to snore and no longer reacts to having the eyelashes lightly brushed with a finger, it is time to deepen the anaesthetic. From now on the patient's chin needs to be supported, to stop the tongue rolling back and obstructing the airway. Get the anaesthetist or one of the trained staff to demonstrate to you the correct method of doing this. *Maintenance of a clear airway is now everyone's top priority.* Having put the syringes aside, the anaesthetist will now relieve you of this task. He or she will then apply the face mask, allowing the patient to breathe pure oxygen initially, and then gradually adding nitrous oxide and a volatile anaesthetic agent. You can regulate the flowmeters for him or her.

Now that the airway is safe, you can turn your attention to the rest of the patient's body. In this extremely relaxed state the body is floppy, and the patient's arms in particular are prone to falling over the edge of the operating table. If left like this, the continuous pressure of the table could cause irreparable damage to the brachial plexus, not to mention pressure sores. So secure the patient's arms with padded arm supports, and straighten the legs, adding heel supports.

If the operative procedure is to be short, the anaesthetist will next insert the oral airway, to be used in conjunction with the mask. Lubricate one of an appropriate size. The anaesthetist may also wish to use a harness to support the chin, thus releasing his or her hands of the chore. As the anaesthetist lifts the patient's head, you can slip this underneath and secure the straps on the hooks on the mask. Never try and move the patient's head without the anaesthetist's knowledge and supervision; you may compromise the airway or make the patient cough.

Intubation

If the patient is to undergo a long operation where relaxation or paralysis of a major muscular structure is desirable, such as of the hip or the abdominal muscles, the anaesthetist will intubate. You can be standing by with the tray of instruments to assist. Firstly, the anaesthetist will need the laryngoscope to visualize the glottis, epiglottis and the vocal cords. If he or she likes to use a local anaesthetic spray, this will be next. There are two reasons for doing this. One is to prevent laryngospasm, and the other is

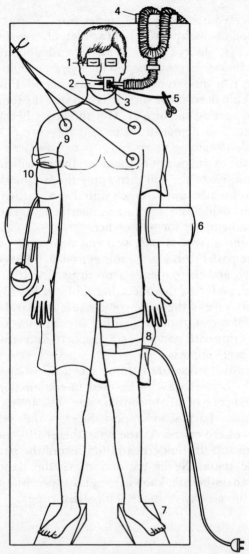

Fig. 5.2   The intubated patient ready for theatre. **1** Eye strapping. **2** Gauze roll tied around endotracheal tube. **3** Gauze under metal connections. **4** Tubing support. **5** Pilot tube occluded by an artery forceps. **6** Arm supports with soft padding beneath. **7** Heel supports. **8** Diathermy pad supported by Velcro strapping. **9** ECG electrodes. **10** Blood pressure cuff.

to prevent fluctuations in blood pressure and cardiac arrhythmias, which can result from interference with the very sensitive vocal cords.

Now the endotracheal tube can be passed. The anaesthetist will already have indicated to you which of the selection of tubes he or she wishes to use, and you will have given it a good coating of lubricant gel. Normally an introducer is not used, but it should be available to give greater rigidity to the tube in difficult cases. The anaesthetist aims to slide the tube down between the cords, and must check straight away that it is in the right place, inflating the lungs and not the stomach! To do this the endotracheal tube must be connected to the anaesthetic circuit. So while the anaesthetist is intubating, you can remove the face mask from the circuit and connect the catheter mount, which fits on to the end of the tube, in its place. The anaesthetist can then hand-ventilate the patient using the squeezy reservoir bag, and listen with a stethoscope for breath sounds. If the endotracheal tube is in the wrong place, the whole procedure will have to be repeated. Remember that until the tube is in the right place, the patient is not breathing or getting any oxygen to the brain, so speed is of the essence. This is why all the connections must be carefully checked beforehand.

Once the tube is in the right place, the cuff must be inflated. This anchors the tube in position and provides an airtight seal so that no aspirate from the stomach can enter the lungs. Fill the 20 ml syringe with air and pass this to the anaesthetist, shortly followed by the artery forceps to occlude the pilot tube. Once the anaesthetist is happy that all is well, the tube will need to be secured externally, using a length of gauze roll or strapping. Make sure that metal connectors are supported by gauze and are not directly in contact with the skin, where they are potential sites for diathermy burns or pressure marks. Also check that the circuit is not dragging too heavily on the patient's mouth, traumatizing the lips. Intubation is now complete, and once inside the operating theatre, the anaesthetist will connect the circuit up to the mechanical ventilator to take over control of the patient's breathing.

Nasal intubation

This is carried out when surgical access to the mouth is necessary – most commonly for dental operations. The steps of the procedure are much the same. The laryngoscope is inserted through the mouth as usual, but the tube is passed through the nose and guided down between the vocal cords using a pair of Magill intubation forceps. There are a few differences between nasal and endotracheal tubes. Firstly a narrower lumen is necessary, as the nostril gives smaller access to the trachea than via the mouth. Secondly, they need to be longer, as they have further to reach. As a rough guide, a size 7 is normally used for a woman, and a size 8 for a man. Nasal tubes are also not cuffed. Instead, the lumen of the pharynx is packed with a length of damp gauze roll, again using the Magill forceps. Care must be taken to ensure that this is removed postoperatively.

The tube is normally supported by strapping on the patient's face and a Velcro fastening head band, which helps to take the weight of the circuit. Again, metal connectors should be padded with gauze, and special care is needed to protect the eyes from corneal abrasions. A piece of light strapping, such as Transpore, over the lashes of the closed eyes should be sufficient protection. (Remember to leave one edge doubled over for easy removal.)

One essential piece of equipment which must always be at hand throughout nasal intubation is a small dental suction head or suction catheter. The normal sized suction head will be too big to give adequate clearance of the airway.

CRASH INDUCTION OR SELLICK'S MANOEUVRE

This is an emergency measure used when a patient has not been starved, or where there is excess pressure on the stomach, as in pregnancy or a hiatus hernia with reflux symptoms. When this patient is intubated, one of the induction drugs the anaesthetist gives is a muscle relaxant. Surgical access to the abdomen is then possible, but the patient will require artificial ventilation of the lungs. Relaxation does present one major problem however, which is that in such a state the patient may regurgitate and inhale the contents of the stomach, since there is now no cough reflex to keep the airway clear. The patient could asphyxiate and die as a result, or be left with a serious chest infection. This risk is present for every patient, but is minimized by preoperative starving. For those needing emergency surgery who will not have been starved, or for pregnant women needing a caesarean section in whom the enlarged uterus presses on the stomach, or for the patient with the hiatus hernia, this risk is much greater.

Sellick's manoeuvre is employed in these instances. The cricoid cartilage is compressed during induction; this occludes the oesophagus by pressing it back against the cervical vertebrae. The pressure must be maintained until the cuff of the endotracheal tube has been adequately inflated and secured. The lungs are now sealed off, so that no acid gastric contents can enter.

If the anaesthetist plans to use this manoeuvre, you must explain to the patient that he or she will feel someone pressing on the neck as he or she goes off to sleep. Give reassurance that this is normal procedure. Have the anaesthetist show you the exact spot where you are expected to press before induction begins. Do not try and get involved with the other equipment now: the anaesthetist can manage alone with the intubation tray. Just concentrate on pressing: your patient's life may depend upon it. For a better understanding of the effectiveness of this procedure, check the position of the cricoid cartilage in your anatomy book.

Now that the anaesthetic is under control, there are still a few things to be done before entering the theatre. Monitoring devices need to be attached. Three disposable electrodes are applied to the body in order to give an ECG trace. They are placed one on the anterior aspect of each shoulder, and one just below the left breast, near the apex of the heart. These connect to a bundle of three leads, which are colour-coded; usually red connects to the right shoulder, yellow to the left and black to the lower electrode. A blood pressure cuff should also be in place. The patient may now need to be positioned for surgery (see Chapter 2 for a description of the different table positions). Keep prevention of pressure sores, diathermy burns and damage to nerve tissue uppermost in your mind. Also think of preserving the patient's dignity; keep the theatre gown in place until surgery is just about to commence. Do not leave the patient unnecessarily exposed.

CATHETERIZATION

This is often carried out in the anaesthetic room, where surgery indicates the need for it. Here at least is one familiar procedure, and one which you may be happy to undertake, provided the sex of the patient is appropriate. If you have not catheterized before here is a good chance to learn, under the supervision of a trained nurse. If you are assisting, you need to position the patient first.

Ensure that the operating gown is tucked well away, to give good access to the urethra. Women's legs need to be bent at the knee simultaneously, and allowed to abduct, so that they rest apart. Placing the soles of the feet together is often adequate to maintain this position. Elderly patients, or those with poor joint movement, may need their legs supported throughout the procedure.

Ensure that there is a good light on the perineum, and then you can open the catheterization pack and other sterile articles on to a clean trolley. You will also need to pour the antiseptic lotion. Readjust the patient's position once the catheter is secure and draining.

ENTERING THE THEATRE

Now you are ready to transfer the patient into the operating theatre. You want to ensure a rapid transfer, so that the patient is disconnected from the ventilator for the shortest space of time possible. Check that there are no impediments to your path before the anaesthetist disconnects the circuit in the anaesthetic room. Intravenous infusions must be taken down from their stands; make sure that the table brake is off, the theatre doors are open, and that the anaesthetic machine in theatre is standing ready.

Your first priority is to connect the patient up to the new circuit immediately. Help the anaesthetist to re-set the flowmeters at the required rate. Put the table brake back on, and then get your monitoring equipment in working order. Switch on the ECG machine and connect the leads so that a satisfactory trace is visible. Connect the blood pressure cuff to the sphygmomanometer. Hang the intravenous infusions on stands at the head end of the table, and if the anaesthetist particularly wants access to an infusion site, it is a good idea to insert an arm board, to which the extended arm can be lightly strapped or bandaged. If a catheter is in situ, hang the bag on a stand at the foot of the table, where the anaesthetist will be able to see it once the sterile drapes are in position.

Now that your patient is safe and comfortable, make sure that the anaesthetist is. If he or she is holding the patient's jaw, he or she is not able to move around freely to get all that is necessary, so you are being relied on heavily. Find a stool for the anaesthetist to sit on, and ensure access to the patient's anaesthetic and prescription charts. (Place the other notes and x-rays in a place where the surgical team also have access to them.) The other equipment which the anaesthetist needs is the tray of induction drugs used in the anaesthetic room, and also the intubation equipment. Bring these through and place them on the anaesthetic machine, where the anaesthetist can reach them easily. The other essential piece of equipment is a working sucker at hand. Ask if there is anything else the anaesthetist needs.

DURING SURGERY

The anaesthetist has three major responsibilities during surgery. Firstly, he or she must maintain a clear airway and adequately ventilate the lungs. Secondly, he or she must maintain a good, regular cardiac output and minimize the effects of surgical shock by administering pain relief and replacing lost body fluids. Thirdly, he or she must keep the patient in a state of anaesthesia, so that the latter is unaware of the surgery. A fourth responsibility could be added to this list, and that is meeting the needs of the surgeon. Sometimes extra muscle relaxation or a lower blood pressure facilitates surgery.

During a long operation there is plenty of opportunity for you to learn how all of these requirements are met. Observe how the patient's condition is monitored and how drugs and intravenous fluids are used; above all, ask the anaesthetist lots of questions. Once you have prepared the anaesthetic room for the next patient, there is not normally a lot you need to be doing. Your role is now to be available and able to respond when help is needed. It is vital for the anaesthetist to have assistance throughout the operation, whether simply to collect extra drugs or units of blood and equipment, or to assist in case of emergency.

REVERSAL OF THE ANAESTHETIC AND EXTUBATION

At the end of a long operation where the patient has been intubated, the anaesthetic needs to be reversed before the tube can be taken out. When you see that the surgeon is preparing to close the wound, you can start to prepare the necessary equipment. This is when the intubation tray is needed again. In particular, the anaesthetist will need the laryngoscope and the 20 ml syringe again, the face mask and angled connector used in induction and a lubricated airway of appropriate size. Make sure that working suction equipment is also still at hand.

Reversing the anaesthetic means giving a drug which is an antidote to the muscle relaxant (see above). Any volatile agent used will have gradually been tailed off, giving a smaller and smaller concentration, as the anaesthetist observed the operation drawing to a close. Analgesics, other than nitrous oxide, will have been carefully used, bearing in mind the estimated length of the operation, to give a fine balance of some postoperative analgesia without compromising the patient's ability to make a quick recovery. (Occasionally, however, drugs have to be administered to reverse the effect of opiates, so that patients do not have depressed respiration.) Have the appropriate reversal drugs at hand, along with syringes, needles and drug labels. The anaesthetist will inject these intravenously as the wound is being closed, and then hand-ventilate the patient again.

When the patient begins to cough and struggle, indicating that reflexes have returned, it is time to remove the endotracheal tube. Before this is done, have your empty 20 ml syringe ready, so that the anaesthetist can let down the cuff, and remove any strapping or gauze roll securing the tube. Make sure that you remove any eye covering now, as it is frightening to wake up and be unable to see. The suction must be switched on now, so that immediately the tube is out, you can hand the anaesthetist the laryngoscope followed by the suction head to clear any secretions from the airway. Next you will need the oral airway, and you can attach the face mask back on to the circuit, in case the anaesthetist wishes to give more oxygen. Monitoring equipment which the anaesthetist no longer requires can now also be removed, such as the disposable electrodes and the blood pressure cuff. Finally, you can help to lift and position the patient, usually on the side in the recovery position, on the bed or trolley. Before the anaesthetist finally disappears to recovery with the patient, make sure that he or she has signed for any controlled drugs used.

CLEARING UP

There is a fair amount of clearing up to do at the end of an operation. Suction bottles must be washed and replaced, and fresh tubing and suction heads put out ready for the next patient.

(Remember to check the function again.) All syringes, needles and left-over drugs must be discarded. If any of these are controlled drugs, you must get a trained nurse to witness this and record the wastage in the controlled drugs register. Disposable equipment, such as electrodes and some endotracheal tubes, can simply be thrown out. The rubber masks and harnesses should be scrubbed under hot running water, unless the patient was known to have an infection, in which case they should be washed in detergent, dried and then autoclaved. Laryngoscope blades, connectors for the endotracheal tubes, catheter mounts and artery forceps should also be scrubbed in a detergent solution, and autoclaved if possible because of the increased risk of contracting blood-borne diseases these days. Oral airways and non-disposable endotracheal tubes are normally sterilized by the Theatre Sterile Supplies Unit (TSSU), but they should be given an initial scrub and soak in an antiseptic solution.

EPIDURAL, SPINAL AND CAUDAL ANAESTHESIA

These are all forms of specialized local anaesthetics which in some circumstances can be used as an alternative to the general anaesthetic. First of all some definitions.

For an *epidural*, local anaesthetic is introduced to the area just before, or outside, the dura mater, where it can act on nerve roots entering and leaving the spinal cord.

A *spinal* anaesthetic is where a deeper injection of the drug is given. The injection pierces all the layers covering the spinal cord, but at a site below the level to which the cord extends. (The cord could easily be damaged by a needle, with disastrous results for the patient.) The anaesthetic drug is thus mixed into the cerebrospinal fluid.

A *caudal* is a specialized type of epidural anaesthetic. The drug is injected into the small aperture of the base of the spine at sacral level. It is particularly useful for pain relief during and after surgery around the perineum, such as in haemorrhoidectomy and circumcision. Often it is used in conjunction with rather than instead of, a general anaesthetic.

All of these anaesthetics work by anaesthetizing nerve roots below the level at which they were injected. They also produce muscle relaxation, and through their effect on the sympathetic nervous system, dilation of blood vessels and a low blood pressure in the area of surgery. These are excellent conditions for the surgeon to work in. Vasopressor drugs, such as adrenaline, must always be at hand however, and intravenous access established before the anaesthetic begins, so that any severe drop in blood pressure can be immediately counteracted.

Everything below the point of injection is anaesthetized, while all above is working normally. This provides the clue to the best uses of these anaesthetics. Spontaneous breathing is preserved, so it is ideal for the elderly with chronic lung diseases, considered unfit for general anaesthesia. Obese patients are good candidates too, as they more commonly develop postoperative chest infections. Large, muscular men undergoing operations such as prostatectomy or haemorrhoidectomy, who would normally require high doses of muscle relaxant, can also benefit. These types of anaesthetic are becoming more common, and particularly so in obstetrics, where women require pain relief during labour, but also wish to be fully awake and alert when their child is born. Prolonged postoperative or post-labour pain relief can also be achieved by the same method, if the access catheter is left in place.

The anaesthetic drugs commonly used in this way are lignocaine, Nupercaine and Marcain. They are available in different strength solutions, and come in sterilized, pre-packed ampoules.

These anaesthetics are administered under aseptic conditions. If the anaesthetist plans to use one of these methods, he or she will scrub up, gown and glove as for an operation. You will need to clean a trolley and open the appropriate sterile pack. This should contain the necessary instruments and swabs for cleansing the skin, the linen for draping and a selection of glass syringes. You will need to add the skin cleansing lotion, a spinal needle, ordinary needles for drawing up the drug, the drug itself and a spinal catheter, if one is to be left in place so that the anaesthetic can be topped up. Also have some sleek strapping available to anchor the catheter in place. Have the anaesthetist tell you exactly what is wanted before he or she scrubs up.

Patients need careful preparation. Ensure that the anaesthetic room is warm enough, as their back will need to be exposed, and make sure that it is as quiet as possible. Most departments have 'Patient Awake' signs which can be displayed outside the theatre, to remind others passing of the need for quiet. The anaesthetist should have fully explained the procedure to the patient on the ward. You can reinforce this information, reminding the patient of the different steps as they occur.

The patient should be positioned lying on the side, or else sitting up and leaning forward. A cross-table with a pillow on top makes the ideal support for the latter position. The patient's back must be fully exposed. Once the anaesthetist has everything he or she wants on the trolley, you should stand on the side the patient is facing to give comfort and support. Observe your patient carefully throughout the procedure. Watch out especially for signs of breathlessness or shock.

Once the catheter is in place and has been securely fastened with sleek strapping, the patient should be carefully laid on the side, if not in this position already. He or she must not be allowed to sit up again until the effects of the anaesthetic have worn off.

Once the anaesthetic is working, remember that although the patient is awake, the lower limbs and body are anaesthetized. So take the same care in moving and positioning this patient for surgery as you would with one who had had a general anaesthetic. Think of preventing pressure sores, diathermy burns and nerve damage due to pressure from parts of the table.

When the operation is underway, you can sit on a stool by the patient's head where you can continue to give quiet support and observe the patient's general condition. Immediately report to the surgeon, or to the anaesthetist if available, any untoward symptoms or signs that the anaesthetic is not working. In recovery, observations of blood pressure, pulse, respirations and the patient's colour will continue to be made frequently, and special attention should be paid to preventing over-distension of the bladder which, of course, the patient will not feel.

Local anaesthesia

This is where only the site of operation is anaesthetized. Local anaesthesia can be administered in two different ways – by direct application to mucous membranes or by injection. The latter is the commonest method.

This is done as part of the sterile operative procedure. All the necessary syringes and needles are put on to the scrub nurse's trolley, and he or she draws up the local anaesthetic from sterile ampoules offered by the circulating assistant. As anaesthetic nurse, this leaves you free to give the patient your undivided attention.

Make sure that the patient is comfortable on the operating

table, with enough pillows and arm supports if these help. Make sure the patient is warm enough. An anaesthetic screen should be in position, so that the patient will not see the operation; when this is covered by a sterile drape, ensure that the patient's face is uncovered and that he or she is breathing easily. As always, protect the patient's dignity, and only expose the site of operation when the surgeon is ready to begin. Sit with the patient in a convenient position, out of the surgeon's way, and offer quiet support. Remember that if you felt frightened and apprehensive upon entering the operating suite, what must it be like for the patient? He or she has entered this alien environment fully conscious, and is to undergo surgery without being put to sleep! One way of helping the patient is to give orientation in time, providing progress reports throughout the operation. Knowing that 'the lump is out now' and 'the surgeon just has to put a few stitches in now' often helps to make the whole thing bearable, setting a time limit to the duration of discomfort. Observe the patient constantly for signs of pain and distress; the surgeon can always inject more local anaesthetic.

The most commonly used local anaesthetics are lignocaine and Marcain. They are available in different strength solutions, and are sometimes mixed with adrenaline. This prolongs the effect of the anaesthetic, preventing it from being absorbed by the body too quickly, and also reduces bleeding in the area, making the surgeon's job easier. Such a mixture must never be injected into a digit or ear lobe, tip of the nose or the penis, however, as there is a risk of subsequent ischaemia or gangrene developing as a result of the vasoconstrictor effect.

Nerve blocks

These are specific local anaesthetics aimed at blocking particular nerve pathways. A common one you might meet is the *paravertebral* block, where an injection is made between the ribs to block nerve pathways as they leave the vertebral column. This anaesthetizes the chest or abdominal wall, depending on the level of injection, on that side. The *brachial plexus* block is also fairly common. Here, the arm is anaesthetized by injecting at the root of the neck, above the collar bone.

Intravenous injection

A most effective way of anaesthetizing a limb is by intravenous injection, which suffuses the whole limb. To do this, the blood supply to that limb has to be temporarily isolated from that of the rest of the body. This procedure is commonly referred to as a regional anaesthetic or Bier's block, and is perhaps most often used for manipulation of fractures of the wrist. The patient's blood pressure needs to be measured before starting, so that throughout the procedure checks can be made to ensure that the tourniquet cuff is kept at a level above that of the patient's systolic pressure. This ensures that there is no leakage of local anaesthetic into the general circulation.

The limb should be elevated and then a tourniquet, with orthopaedic wool padding underneath, is applied around the top, where the limb joins the trunk. The limb then needs to be exsanguinated, using a special exsanguination device or an Esmarch bandage. The tourniquet is then inflated. The blood supply to the limb has now been isolated from the rest of the body. The local anaesthetic can be injected, and the operative procedure may commence.

Afterwards, the tourniquet should be released very slowly and the patient observed closely, as a large bolus of local anaesthetic is now being released into the general circulation. The patient should rest for at least 15–20 minutes before trying to get up and move. Observations of the limb should also be made following the procedure to ensure that there is a good circulation. The site of the tourniquet, and how long it was in position, should be recorded in the nursing notes.

CHILDREN IN THE ANAESTHETIC ROOM

Paediatric anaesthesia is a specialized subject which this book will not attempt to explain. Instead, some of the differences and the important considerations relating to children will be highlighted.

If you do get the chance to see children or neonates anaesthetized, you will realize that the equipment used is rather different, to accommodate the differences in their anatomy. Everything is on a very small scale.

It is best if you simply stand back and observe how the

anaesthetist works, helped by a trained nurse or ODA. If you help to prepare the anaesthetic room, although this sounds obvious, remember to *think small*! Check that there is a paediatric or dental suction head ready for use, and that small pieces of strapping or bandage are available, for example.

When children come to the operating department, they are almost always accompanied by a parent. Therefore, two people here are in need of your support, and quite often it will be the parent who needs more reassurance than the premedicated child.

Children are normally anaesthetized by inhalation, in order to avoid nasty injections. If the child is already sleeping peacefully on arrival, the transition to the anaesthetized state can be simple and untraumatic. Remember that peace and quiet in the anaesthetic room are extremely important when it comes to children. Disturb the child as little as possible. A frightened, screaming child is very difficult to settle again, and makes a stressful atmosphere for both parent and staff.

One very important fact to remember when dealing with children or babies is that they lose body heat far more rapidly than adults. Make sure the anaesthetic room is nice and warm before the child arrives, and prevent heat loss by keeping all the doors closed. You will notice how the trained staff will often put a warming mattress covered with gamgee on to the table before induction, and perhaps wrap the child in gamgee, ready-warmed in the heated lotions cabinet. For neonates, tin foil swaddlers are often used.

To recap, when dealing with children or babies, an extra-peaceful, extra-warm atmosphere is needed. Think on a small scale when preparing equipment, and be prepared to welcome and comfort the parent as well as the child.

Further reading

Atkinson, R.S. *et al.* (1982). *A Synopsis of Anaesthesia: general anaesthesia, regional anaesthesia and intensive therapy*, 9th ed. Bristol: J. Wright.

Bonner M. (1986). Can my friend go with me? *Nursing Times/Nursing Mirror*, **82**, 40, p. 75.

Shergold L. (1986). Epidural and spinal anaesthetics. *Nursing Times/Nursing Mirror*, **82**, 27, p. 44.

Siddall W. (1982). The care of children requiring surgery. *NAT News*, **19**(6), pp. 22–4.

Anaesthetics 65

Taylor J. (1986). What did he say nurse? *NAT News*, **23**(8), pp. 14–17.
Ward C. S. (1985). *Anaesthetic Equipment; Physical Principles and Maintenance*, 2nd ed. London: Balliere-Tindall, 1985.

6

Instruments

If the person on the street was asked about the job of theatre nurse, I'm sure most would say that it consisted solely of passing instruments to the surgeon; that, and mopping the surgeon's brow! Although it is important to know which are the right tools for the job in hand, and how these should be prepared and maintained, instrumentation is only one aspect of the work of the theatre nurse. For the student nurse it is a far less important aspect than grasping the essentials of the overall care of the surgical patient. This chapter aims to give a brief and simple introduction to the subject, and to put it in its true perspective.

When you first enter the operating department you may be forgiven for thinking that you will have to learn all the names of the instruments. Many students mistakenly believe that this is expected of them. Where on earth does one begin? There are so many different instruments, and all with such complicated, forgettable names! A proficient scrub nurse in action is an awesome sight, one which you could never dream of emulating. But take comfort. Most theatre nurses would disagree that this is the most difficult part of the job.

Instruments can easily be separated into different categories, according to their function. An example of a category would be 'artery forceps' or 'dissecting forceps'. Once they are thus classified, the variety within each category appears much less daunting. The number of different possible categories is in fact very small. Understanding the function of an instrument is far more important and useful than knowing its specific name.

If you plan to work in the operating department as a staff nurse, you will gradually learn all the specific names of instruments – even all the double-barrelled ones – and you will learn by an easy process of absorption as you use the instruments constantly. Indeed you will soon also learn that many surgeons don't know the specific names for instruments either. A lot of them make up their own names or else use a blanket term such as 'clip' for a whole variety of different artery forceps. If you ever spend time working in other hospitals, you will also realize that different places often have different names for the same instruments. So you can see that while knowing specific names is attractive to the perfectionist, and indeed provides some interesting clues to the historical development of surgical instruments, it is by no means a necessity for you at the present.

To illustrate my point, let us now take a look at some categories of instruments. Here is a list of the contents of a large general surgery set. Firstly, the different categories are listed, and then each category will be examined more closely.

GENERAL SET

Categories

1   2 7" Rampley spongeholders.
    2 9½" Rampley spongeholders.
2   6 Mayo towel clips
3   1 no. 3 BP handle.
    1 no. 4 BP handle.
    1 no. 5 BP handle.
4   Nurses ligature/stitch scissors.
    1 6½" Mayo scissors – curved.
    1 7" McIndoe scissors.
    1 9" Lobectomy scissors (Nelson's).
5   1 6" Gillie's toothed dissecting forceps.
    1 7" Lane's toothed dissecting forceps.
    1 6" McIndoe's non-toothed dissecting forceps.
    1 7" Non-toothed dissecting forceps.
    1 7" DeBakey non-toothed dissecting forceps.
    1 10" DeBakey non-toothed dissecting forceps.
6   5 5" Dunhill artery forceps – curved.
    10 7" Spencer Wells artery forceps – straight.
    5 7¾" Lahey artery forceps.
    5 8" Moynihan cholecystectomy forceps.
    5 9" Roberts artery forceps - curved.
7   2 6" Allis tissue forceps.
    2 6" Babcock tissue forceps.
    2 6" Lane's tissue forceps.
8   2 Medium Langenbeck retractors 1¾" × ½".
    2 Morris double-ended retractors.

    1 Guy's hospital pattern liver retractor.
    1 3″ Deaver retractor.
    1 Ogilvie retractor.
    1 Traver's self-retaining retractor.
    1 Balfour retractor and Doyen blade.
 9 2 6″ Mayo needleholders.
    1 8½″ Crile-wood needleholder.
    1 9½″ Crile-wood needleholder.
10 1 6″ Remington diathermy forceps.
    1 8″ Remington diathermy forceps.
    1 Diathermy lead.
    1 Quiver.
11 1 Poole's suction end and guard.
    1 Yankaur sucker.
    (1 Zimmer bag clip.)

1. Spongeholding forceps

Use: An instrument upon which to mount skin-cleaning sponges
or else small swabs for use in deep wounds. The forceps are made
in different lengths; the shorter ones for cleaning the skin and the
longer ones for the deep work. They are shaped and operated
like scissors but instead of blades they have blunt, loop-shaped
surfaces at the tips, with an inner grid pattern to give a better
grip. They have a ratchet half-way down, which will lock when
the forceps are in the closed position. This prevents small swabs
being lost inside the wound.

Mounting spongeholding forceps

To mount skin-cleaning sponges, open the ratchet of the instrument and align the tops half-way up the length of the sponge,
then close the ratchet. This gives a nice firm grip, while leaving
plenty of the sponge free at the top for the surgeon to clean with.
    Mounting swabs takes a little more practice. Again, open the
ratchet and align the forceps tips half-way up the short side of
the folded 3″ × 4″ swab. Do not close the ratchet, but allow. the
tips to touch, so gripping the swab. Wind the rest of the length
around the tips and finally catch the loose end between them
before closing the ratchet. This is commonly referred to as a 'swab
on a stick'.

2. Towel clips

Use: for securing the drapes and anchoring other equipment to them, such as a diathermy lead. These are small instruments with curved blades and sharp pointed ends. Some are scissor-shaped with a ratchet, and some are shaped like a figure of 8, and work by spring action.

3. Knife (Bard–Parker) handles

Use: Handles on which to mount surgical blades for incising tissue. The handles come in different numbered sizes – 3, 4 and 5 are the most commonly used. You will find the numbers etched on the handles, towards the rounded base.

No. 3 is a short, thin handle upon which to mount the more delicate range of blades. This combination of shortness and fineness means that a no. 3 handle is suitable for superficial surgery confined to a small area, for example removing facial lesions or releasing trapped nerves in the hand. The most commonly used blades here will be a no. 10 and a no. 15. You may also come across a no. 11 blade, which is sharp-pointed and used for arteriotomy, i.e. incising blood vessels. (Apologies for all these numbers, but this is how the manufacturers differentiate between the blades and how they are commonly referred to in the theatre. To see the differences in the shapes of blades, look at the illustrations on the sides of the manufacturers' boxes.)

No. 4 is a broader, slightly longer handle, to take blades used for making longer and deeper incisions, such as in abdominal or hip operations. Blade nos 20–23 are the commonest.

No. 5 is a very long, fine handle. As you might expect, this is used for delicate dissection inside a deep wound. It takes the same blades as a no. 3 handle.

Mounting blades

Grip the blade firmly near the top, using a needleholder with a ratchet. Align the bottom slant of the blade with its corresponding line on the handle. Slide the raised groove at the top of the handle into the cut-out groove in the blade. The blade should now be firmly in position (Fig. 6.1). Never handle blades with your fingers, they are very sharp!

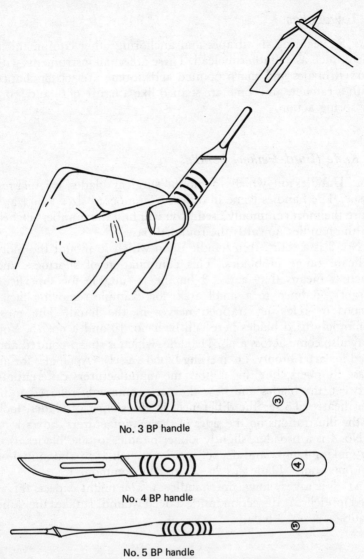

No. 3 BP handle

No. 4 BP handle

No. 5 BP handle

Fig. 6.1 Knife (BP) handles, and how to mount them

Removing blades

Turn the mounted handle over so that the side you used for aligning the blade to the handle is facing downwards. Hold the handle at an angle, with the blade lower than the handle, and make sure no one is standing directly in front of you. (Sometimes blades spring off and anyone nearby could be cut.) Now take the ratcheted needleholder, and grip the blade where it adjoins the handle. Pull firmly downwards, and the blade will come off.

4. Scissors

Use: For dissecting tissue, and cutting sutures, ties and dressing material. Here at least is a familiar instrument. The scissors in the general set vary in length and heaviness. As with the knives, the different lengths of scissors indicate the depth at which they can be used. The heaviness or coarseness of a pair of scissors indicates the type of tissue or material they are suitable for cutting. For instance, fine scissors will be used for cutting peritoneum, whereas heavy scissors are needed to cut tough layers of muscle. Scissors also vary in that their blades may be curved or straight, and their tips sharp or round-ended (often referred to as 'blunt'). Round-ended scissors are most commonly used as they are less likely to traumatize adjacent tissues. Straight, round-ended scissors are used to cut sutures, ties and dressings, while a surgeon will always dissect with curved round-ended scissors. The curve prevents trauma to adjacent tissue by making the cut more limited in length and more precise. It also helps the surgeon follow the natural curve of bodily structures, which on the whole are rounded.

From time to time you may also come across scissors with angled blades and sharp tips; these are arteriotomy scissors.

5. Dissecting forceps

Use: For gripping and handling tissue. These are the V-shaped, tweezer-like forceps used constantly throughout an operation. Like the scissors, they vary in length and heaviness, for the same reasons. If you are working in a deep dark hole you need long forceps; short ones won't reach! If you are trying to grip a thick layer of abdominal fat, fine forceps are useless, as would be a heavy pair for delicate facial work. (By now you will be getting the hang of the simple logic which governs instrument design; and in time, should the surgeon not specify, you will be able to make correct decisions about which variety of instrument to hand over for which job.)

The other thing to mention about dissecting forceps is that some have teeth and some don't. Delicate tissues would be

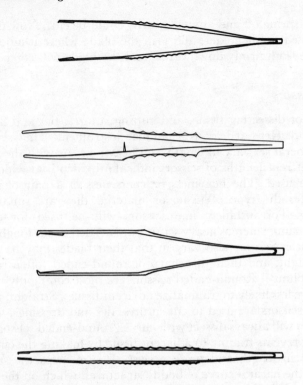

Fig. 6.2   Dissecting forceps

punctured and damaged by teeth, therefore they must be handled by non-toothed forceps. Coarser tissues are much more easily handled and not harmed by a toothed grip. In general, non-toothed forceps are used for handling internal organs, blood vessels, nerves and peritoneum. Toothed forceps are used on muscle, fat and skin (Fig. 6.2).

6. Artery forceps

Use: These are used primarily for occluding blood vessels. Bleeding vessels can then be tied off or diathermized, so that there is haemostasis, i.e. no further bleeding.

Artery forceps also have several secondary uses. Small ones can be used as markers on the ends of sutures or swab tapes, larger ones for mounting ties to be passed around deep bleeding points or for mounting dissecting swabs. Artery forceps are used also for gripping and lifting layers of tissue to facilitate suturing or dissection.

They often appear to be the most confusing instruments to learn as there are so many of them in a set, and they all look so alike. However they follow the same logic in design as everything else. They vary in length and heaviness, and in whether or not they are curved or straight. Generally speaking, the longer they are, the more fully curved they are, as this makes them easier to manoeuvre inside a deep wound.

On the subject of curves, let us deal with some terms you may hear used. All of the artery forceps and scissors in this set could be referred to as being 'curved on flat'. This simply means that they curve upwards from their flat top surface. You may come across some artery forceps which are termed 'curved on the side', but these are relatively rare, used mainly in neurosurgery (Fig. 6.3).

All artery forceps have ratchets, so that once applied to a bleeding vessel they will not slip. There is usually some kind of grid pattern on the inner surfaces of the tips, to enhance this grip. Strictly speaking they do not have teeth, for the same reasons that some dissecting forceps do not have them. (You may however come across Kochers artery forceps which do have teeth. These are used mainly in orthopaedic surgery, and really to term them artery forceps is something of a misnomer.)

7. Tissue forceps

Use: for gripping and handling tissue. Tissue forceps have much the same function as dissecting forceps, but with two distinctive features. They all have ratchets, so that once applied to tissue there is no need for the operator to keep up continued manual pressure, and they have scissor-like handles. They are in fact rather like artery forceps in appearance, obeying the same rules in length and heaviness, but their tips are very different. They are curved outwards, leaving a gap for some bulk of tissue to be gripped. Some tissue forceps are non-toothed, such as Babcock's, which means that they are suitable for gripping more delicate tissues, such as bowel or vas; and some have teeth, such as Lane's tissue forceps, which are useful for handling large skin flaps.

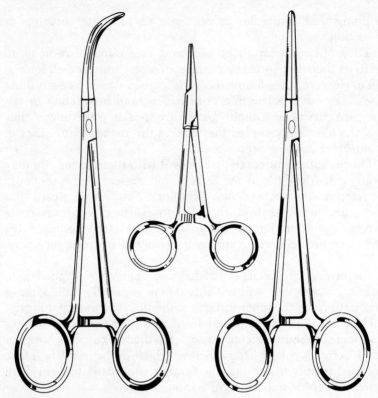

Fig. 6.3   Artery forceps

8. Retractors

Use: For retracting, i.e. pulling back the edges of a wound or internal structure to allow the surgeon better access to the site of operation. Of all the categories of instruments, retractors probably incorporate the most variety, ranging from delicate skin hooks to large liver retractors. Their blades – the part which enters the wound – vary in length and weight. Some have hooks or teeth on them for gripping the more superficial, coarser tissues, while some are blunt. Some blades are flat, i.e. they form a right angle with their handle, with perhaps a small curved lip, while some are more fully curved for deeper work, where they cause less trauma to internal organs. Some are double-ended, which means that they have another blade at the other end, which can be used as a handle for ease of retraction. (If you assist with any abdominal surgery, you will realize what an important feature this is for

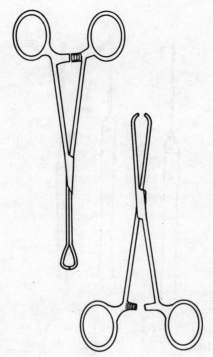

Fig. 6.4   Tissue forceps

your comfort. Retraction can be very hard work!)

Self-retaining retractors make life much easier. No one needs to hold these as once in place they are fixed by means of a ratchet or screw to keep the position of the blades constant (Fig. 6.5).

9. Needleholders

Use: To mount needles on whilst suturing tissue layers. Again needleholders are rather like artery forceps in appearance, but you will notice that there is a much shorter distance between the joint of the instrument and the tips. Needleholders come in different lengths for suturing at different depths, and are fine or heavy according to the type of tissue to be sewn and also the size and shape of the needle to be used. Most have ratchets for a more secure grip on the needle, but there are some without (Fig. 6.6).

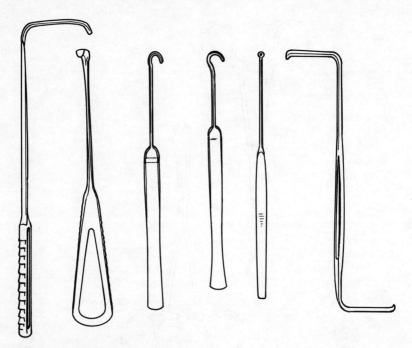

Fig. 6.5 Retractors

10. Diathermy equipment

Use: For cauterizing bleeding vessels and incising tissue.

Diathermy forceps for cauterizing vessels come in two shapes – those of dissecting forceps and those of artery forceps. As such they are subject to the usual design considerations in length, heaviness, shape of curve and in whether they have ratchets or teeth. They are distinguished by their insulated covering for safe handling, and in their point of connection to the diathermy lead.

There is also a straight diathermy 'pencil', to which different tips can be attached. The tip for coagulation is a straight, flat, blunt blade, called a Monel blade. As this instrument has no means to grip a bleeding vessel itself, it has to be used in conjunction with ordinary dissecting or artery forceps. These instruments are touched by the blade, allowing the electric current to pass through them to cauterize the vessels in their grip. Another less common cauterizing attachment which will fit the 'pencil' is a round ball. This is used on fragile tissue, such as the liver, where its smooth, round surface causes minimal trauma.

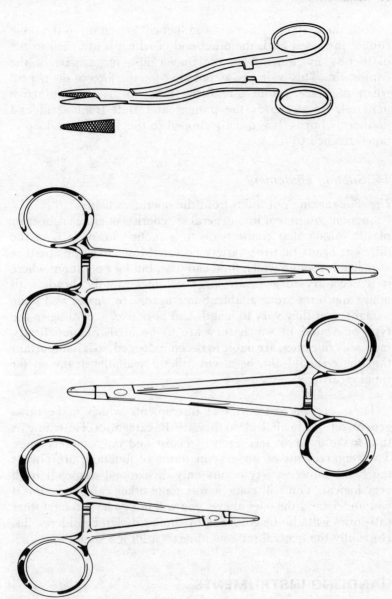

Fig. 6.6 Needleholders

The cutting diathermy attachments also fit on to the 'pencil'. The most common of these is a thin, sharp-pointed needle, but there are also angled needles, and more rarely, wire loops.

Both the diathermy forceps and 'pencil' attach on to the same rubber insulated lead, the other end of which is attached to the diathermy machine. A plastic quiver also forms part of the equipment. This is simply a container for the forceps or 'pencil' when they are not in use. Being made of a non-conductive material, it safeguards the patient and staff from accidental diathermy burns. It is usually clipped to the drapes by a loop of tape attached to it.

11. Suction equipment

Use: For sucking out fluids from the operative field.

Suction equipment in a general set consists of either rubber or plastic tubing that connects on to a suction head. It is in the different heads that the variety occurs. Most have one aperture at the end through which fluid can pass, but for operations where it is necessary to evacuate large volumes rapidly, heads with many apertures are available. Some heads are curved and some straight, and they vary in length and bore size, according to the type of wound in which they are to be used. Suction heads, especially fine ones, are liable to become clogged, so it is important that there should also be a wire stilette available in the set for rapid clearing.

These are the categories of instruments which make up a general set – 11 in all. Indeed they are the categories of instruments that make up most sets, even specialist and microsurgery ones. The requirements of surgery, in terms of function, are always much the same; variety occurs only in size and shape. It is all very logical. You will come across some other categories, but if you understand the ones above, you will not go far wrong. Other categories will also be governed by similar design considerations. Hopefully the general set now appears a lot less daunting!

HANDLING INSTRUMENTS

When you first handle a set of instruments you will probably be feeling nervous, under pressure and ham-fisted. It is not surprising that things tend to get muddled and tangled up together; instruments have a nasty habit of doing this! As far as possible, try and keep the trolley tidy. Return instruments to their original place after use, so that next time you need them, they will be found easily. This also makes it easier to count the instruments at the end of the operation.

Use a damp swab to keep instruments clean. This prevents them becoming sticky and slippery, and more likely to be dropped. Leads should be tangle- and knot-free and securely anchored to the drapes, otherwise they too will slide on to the floor and become unsterile.

Handle instruments by their handles! Try and touch the tips as little as possible, as this is the part which will make most contact with the patient's wound, and therefore the part which should be subject to the least possible contamination.

PASSING INSTRUMENTS

The art of good instrument passing is to place the instrument in the hand of the surgeon, or the assistant, in such a way that it can be used immediately without the operator having to look up. This saves time and the surgeon's concentration will not be broken.

When passing anything with a scissor-type handle, such as scissors, tissue forceps, artery forceps, hold the instrument close to its joint, and place the handle firmly into the surgeon's palm (right palm if right-handed and vice versa if left-handed). If the instrument is curved, the curve should be facing inwards, towards the surgeon's other hand.

When passing dissecting forceps, offer them points down, gripping them by the lower half so that they are closed. The surgeon can then take hold of them at the top, near the joint, and put them straight down into the wound. Offer a swab mounted on forceps in the same way, so that it can be dabbed straight on to the bleeding point.

Retractors should be offered so that the handle goes straight into the surgeons or assistant's hand, and the blade straight into the wound. Again you should hold them at the mid-point.

Needleholders are handed like other instruments with scissor-type handles, making sure that the pointed end of the mounted needle is facing inwards between the surgeon's hands. You should support the end of the length of suture material as you pass it, to prevent it becoming tangled or desterilized (see Chapter 7 for how to mount needles on needleholders).

Knives, as always, should be handled with the greatest care and respect. Grip the handle towards the blade end from above, tilting the blade downwards, with the cutting edge facing the skin. Offered like this, the surgeon can immediately grasp the free end of the handle, and as the knife is drawn away from you there is no danger of you being cut. (Imagine what could happen if you hold the handle from below!)

Practise all of these manoeuvres when you have the chance, preferably with unsterile instruments before you scrub up to assist with an operation. Pass instruments to yourself, one hand to the other, and you will soon become familiar with their feel, and the correct way to hold them for use.

PREPARATION OF INSTRUMENTS FOR SURGERY

Many operating departments now have a Theatre Sterile Supplies Unit (TSSU) which provides an invaluable service in preparing instruments for surgery. Some part of your allocation may be spent here. The instruments they supply to the theatres are washed, overhauled, sterilized and presented in pre-packed metal trays. Once the outer paper cover, which acts as a dust cover, is removed, these can be placed straight on to a clean trolley, ready for use.

Inside the clean preparation room, the inner paper wrapper and the green towel layer are opened to reveal the instruments. These are neatly laid out in a logical order, secured by wire pins, so that minimum handling and rearrangement is required. The trays also contain the patient drapes, swabs, and enough gallipots, kidney dishes, bowls and jugs for the operation.

For general surgery there is usually a choice of three trays. They contain more or less the same instruments – the 11 categories mentioned above – but in different sizes. You can choose between a small, medium or large tray, depending on what type of surgery is to be performed. More specialized trays can be used in conjunction with these, such as chest, vascular or abdominal extras.

Every set contains a check list. This is a very important document, signed by whoever packed the tray, and listing its precise contents. This is retained, and its accuracy double-checked by theatre staff before the operation commences. If correct, it can then be used to check all the instruments again at the end.

The nurse who used it will then sign that everything is present, and send it back to TSSU with the dirty instruments. The check list therefore facilitates the process of locating lost instruments. It can also be used as a means of communication between the theatre and TSSU staff, to indicate the need for instrument repairs.

As the pre-packed tray system has been so widely adopted in this country, many theatre suites are now being built without their own autoclaves. This has meant that a back-up system of pre-packed extra instruments, prepared either singly or in small numbers, has also become necessary. This allows flexibility in modifying the existing trays and also for replacement of contaminated instruments, without having to open a whole new tray.

The advent of the TSSU has freed nurses from many essential, yet strictly non-nursing duties, such as washing instruments and time-consuming maintenance work. TSSU staff now undertake the task of lubricating jointed instruments and applying anti-rust treatments. They check pointed instruments for sharpness, teeth for chips and breaks, and instruments designed to grip for good tip alignment and worn threads. Diathermy equipment is also checked for electrical safety. The TSSU has been a great boon for theatre nurses.

METHODS OF STERILIZATION

Let us first of all define sterility: it is the state where all infective matter has been destroyed, including vegetative micro-organisms, spores and viruses. If the materials from which surgical instruments are made can withstand sterilization, this will be the state of choice prior to surgery.

The most common method of sterilization in all hospitals is that of *moist heat* or *steam under pressure*. It is a method suitable for most equipment used in the operating department: metal instruments, linen, gauze dressings, glass and most plastics. On average the autoclave cycle takes 40 minutes, making it very quick and convenient.

Pre-packed items to be stored on shelves need to be double-wrapped before autoclaving, using either sheets of waterproof paper or paper bags. Large items or trays to be opened straight on to clean trolleys for surgery will need a green towel wrapper inside these also. This layer should give more than ample coverage so that when opened out, the scrub nurse has a large sterile field on which to work. Paper bags should also give good coverage, with space for at least three good folds at the top of the package for safer handling. The packages and trays are secured with autoclave tape and then loaded on to perforated or slatted metal trays.

Once the autoclave has been securely closed and switched on, the first part of its cycle creates a vacuum, removing all the air particles. Steam is then released into the chamber, reaching a temperature of around 134°C for at least 3.5 minutes. The steam is under pressure, and therefore penetrates every single crevice of the packages in the chamber. The final part of the cycle dries the chamber contents.

Before you use any pre-packed item you must double-check it for sterility. The package should be dry and the layers of wrapping intact. The autoclave tape should also have changed colour. If the cycle has been effective, its diagonal stripes will now be dark brown.

If there is an autoclave in your theatre clean preparation room, the articles sterilized here will not need to be wrapped, as the scrub nurse will unload them straight on to the sterile trolley, ready for use. Checking for sterility is slightly more complicated. You have to consult the trace on the disc of graph paper on the front of the machine. This shows the temperature reached inside the chamber and for how long. There are also Browne's tubes – an unfortunate name, since it introduces another colour! – for monitoring heat change. These small glass tubes contain a red liquid. One should be packed inside the autoclave with each load, and at the end of the cycle, if it has been effective, the liquid in the tube will have turned green. All autoclaves, whether in the TSSU or theatre suites, are given regular, routine checks by hospital technicians.

Dry heat

This is a method of sterilization suitable for glass items, sealed tins or jars and very delicate instruments, such as those used in ophthalmic surgery; autoclaving blunts the fine edges more quickly. The cycle entails putting these items into an electric oven for a period of 1 hour at 160°C.

Radiation

This is a commercial method of sterilization, using ionizing radiation, electron beams or gamma irradiation. Familiar articles sterilized in this way are plastic syringes, sutures and urinary catheters.

Ethylene oxide

This method of sterilization is suitable for items that cannot tolerate the high temperature of steam autoclaving, such as delicate plastics, acrylic implant material and electrical leads. The articles in the chamber are heated to only 60°C, with high humidity of 70–80%. For safety's sake, the ethylene oxide is used mixed with an inert gas, such as carbon dioxide. The process is lengthy, taking 3–4 days, since after sterilization, the articles have to be stored on an open shelf to allow the gas to disperse.

This list is not exhaustive but covers the commonest methods of sterilization which you are likely to meet. Sterility is the state of choice for instruments for surgery, but not all can withstand the process, or else the necessary process is complicated and costly. Disinfection therefore still has a place. This destroys vegetative micro-organisms and viruses, but not spores.

DISINFECTION

Chemical disinfection

This is largely used in the preparation of endoscopic equipment for surgery, as it does not harm the delicate fibreoptic material. Glutaraldehyde or Cidex is the most commonly used agent. It is important to follow the manufacturer's instructions when making up and using the solution. Points to check are how long the solution will remain effective for, and how long items need to be immersed before they can be considered disinfected. Instruments need to be thoroughly cleaned and dried before immersion. Check also that they are completely immersed, and that any taps are open, to allow penetration of the inner as well as the outer surface of the instrument. At the end of the disinfection time, they must be thoroughly rinsed with sterile water before use. This removes all traces of the solution from the instruments, which could potentially cause tissue irritation. Most disinfectant solutions can harm the skin, so staff need to take care, and always wear disposable gloves when handling them.

Pasteurization

This is a method of low temperature disinfection, also suitable for endoscopic equipment. The items are immersed in a heated tank of water at 75°C for at least 10 minutes. The same care should be taken to ensure complete cleansing beforehand and complete immersion and contact with inner as well as outer surfaces.

ENDOSCOPY

Endoscopic surgery is increasingly taking the place of open surgery. The benefits are enormous. The patient is far less traumatized and needs a much shorter stay in hospital; savings are made physically, emotionally and economically. You will no doubt see many endoscopic procedures during your time in the operating department, and so a chapter on instruments is not really complete without some explanation of the principles involved.

Simply, endoscopy is a means of inspecting a hollow organ or cavity using an instrument fitted with a light. The scopes themselves vary, ranging from the old-fashioned rigid designs to very sophisticated, expensive, flexible fibreoptic models. Both work on the same principles however, and since not all hospitals have the full range of new scopes, this discussion will focus upon the cystoscope. This is the most commonly used endoscope of all. It has revolutionized genitourinary surgery, making the retropubic prostatectomy largely an operation of the past. The cystoscope allows this to be done equally successfully transurethrally, and with far less trauma. The cystoscope is of rigid design, and is very simply operated (Fig. 6.7).

The instrument comes in various bore sizes, measured in the French gauge (FG). For adults, the normal range of sizes used is 15–21 FG. Women have a smaller urethra than men, and therefore need a smaller bore scope. If additional operating is to be done, as well as simply inspecting the bladder, then a larger size operating cystoscope is needed, ranging up to 26 FG. Every cystoscope has an obturator. This is the rod which fits snugly

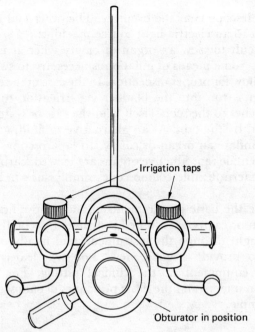

Fig. 6.7 Cystoscope

inside it, with a device to lock the two together. The function of the obturator is to render the cystoscope a round-ended instrument while it is passed into the urethra, thereby causing minimal trauma in passage.

Once the cystoscope is in place, a means of viewing and some light are necessary. The obturator is removed and a telescope is passed inside the cystoscope. Telescopes are delicate instruments which should be handled carefully to prevent damage to the fibreoptics they contain. If you look at the far end of the telescope, away from the eyepiece, you will see the lens and if you look at several telescopes, you will see that the lenses come in various angles. The commonest angles are 0°, which is a flat end, 30° and 70°. These figures are marked on the eyepieces. Normally the surgeon will pass them in this order, so that an ever-widening view of the bladder walls is given.

To pass a telescope, it is first of all necessary to fit it with a connecting piece called a bridge. This has a locking device which fits on to the cystoscope, thus rendering the telescope steady and secure. Light is provided via a fibreoptic light lead, which screws on to the telescope near the eyepiece. The other end of the lead connects on to an electric light source machine.

It is difficult to view an organ or cavity when it is collapsed and hollow. Some means of inflation is necessary to swell out the walls and allow for proper inspection. In the case of the cystoscope, sterile water is run into the bladder via irrigation tubing. This tubing attaches to the scope itself, and the rate of water flow can be regulated by the taps. As an alternative to fluid, gas can also be used to inflate an organ or cavity. In laparoscopy, where the pelvis and female reproductive organs are viewed, carbon dioxide is used. Modern flexible colonoscopes simply suck in air for this purpose.

These are the basic requirements of endoscopy: firstly, access to the organ or cavity via a bored instrument; secondly, a means of passing light through the instrument, and finally, a means of inflation, to provide a good view. You will learn to handle endoscopic equipment in the clinical setting. For now it is important to understand the basic principles of endoscopy, which are very simple.

7

Sutures and wound closure

Why do we close wounds? This seems a ludicrous and unnecessary question, as bodies are naturally intact, but there are several different reasons, some of which you may not have thought of.

As an example, let us take the closure of an abdominal wound, say following bowel resection. First of all the bowel itself needs to be closed. As with all other internal structures, it is closed to prevent spillage of its contents into surrounding cavities, which would result in extreme irritation and infection. In the case of bowel, an unpleasant faecal peritonitis would set in. The bowel is also closed to preserve its function. For peristalsis to occur there needs to be continuity in the muscle fibres, and repairing the visceral tissue helps to prevent the formation of adhesions.

Next the peritoneum is closed. This allows it to continue its protective function, acting as a barrier against infection passing through to the more superficial layers of body tissue and vice versa. Abdominal muscle is also closed to preserve its function in general body movement, and in the prevention of outward herniation of abdominal contents.

Then the subcutaneous layer. This is closed to prevent the formation of pockets of infection, or sinuses, just under the skin. Finally, the skin itself is closed to prevent infection entering the wound, and for cosmetic reasons, to minimize the formation of ugly, fibrous scar tissue.

The cut edges of tissue are sewn, or sutured, together in such a way as to hold them in approximation until natural healing occurs.

FACTORS AFFECTING THE RATE OF WOUND HEALING

The presence of *infection* will always hinder this process considerably. This may be introduced postoperatively by many different routes: an infected lesion elsewhere on the patient's body, contact with body wastes, particularly faeces, seepage from an inadequately closed layer of the wound or from a wound drain. The formation of haematomas below the skin, where wounds have been inadequately drained or haemostasis was not achieved, provides a perfect culture medium for bacteria. Or infection may arise through cross-infection carried by medical or nursing staff, or their equipment. Infection may also have been introduced preoperatively. Foreign bodies left in the wound, such as a swab or an instrument, might be the cause. The instruments used for surgery may have been inadequately sterilized or carelessly contaminated. Whatever the reason for infection of a wound, it will always slow down the natural healing of tissues, and require more careful management. One group of patients needing extra-careful wound management are those who have sustained burns, resulting in skin loss and exposure of deeper tissue.

Good *surgical technique* is vital to promote good wound healing. Asepsis must be rigorously observed and haemostasis achieved before closure of a wound. At the same time, care must be taken to ensure a good blood supply carrying lots of oxygen to the wound edges, which must be well approximated, allowing contact between the capillaries on each side. Tissues should also be handled as little as possible and as gently as possible. This reduces the chances of postoperative bruising and adhesion formation.

The general *health of the patient* plays a major part in dictating the rate of wound healing. Age is an important factor: what may heal in 10 days in a baby may take as many weeks in an old person. The presence of disease is another influential factor. Healthy patients will heal more rapidly than those with diabetes, anaemia or cancer. Indeed treatment for some diseases may also interfere with healing. Patients who have recently undergone radiotherapy, chemotherapy, and especially those whose immune response is suppressed through steroid therapy, will heal more slowly. The nutritional status of patients will similarly have an effect. The malnourished, especially if they lack iron and vitamin C, and the dehydrated will heal more slowly. At the other end of the scale, obese patients will have considerably greater stress on their wounds which is equally detrimental to rapid healing. Wounds inflamed by allergy to sutures, dressing materials or skin preparation lotions will similarly not fare well.

Good *postoperative nursing care*, as you are well aware, also has a powerful potential to influence beneficially the rate of wound healing; this is one factor over which we have complete control. Again, good aseptic technique cannot be stressed enough in wound toilet; special attention should be paid to wounds more vulnerable to contamination, for example, those in the vicinity of a source of infection or on the perineum, where faecal contact is a possibility.

Increasingly the effects of *stress* are also being recognized as interfering with the wound healing process; be it stress directly on the wound, or stress affecting the whole patient – mind and body. Increased levels of adrenaline, secreted in response to stress, interefere with mitosis – the process of division and regeneration of tissue cells. One major stressor, which can easily be relieved, is lack of sleep. Hospital wards are notoriously noisy at night, but with a little care this could be avoided. Indeed it should be avoided, as it is now widely recognized that quicker healing occurs during sleep rather than in waking hours.

Thus many factors influence wound healing, and these need to be taken into account when choosing appropriate regimes of care for individual patients. One aspect of this care is choosing appropriate suture materials.

SUTURES

What is a suture?

It is a strand of material used for tying off blood vessels and sewing tissue edges together. Sutures are used in the same way as when described by Hippocrates, the father of modern medicine. Records of the use of sutures have been found as far back as 2000 BC. Over the years there has been much variety in the materials from which these strands were made: gold, silver and iron wire, silk, silkworm gut, linen, cotton and the tendons and intestines of various animals, to mention just a few.

Today when we use the term *suture*, it is usually understood to refer to a needle and thread together. The strands of material alone are normally termed *ties* or *ligatures*.

At this point let us also deal with two common terms relating to sutures: atraumatic and traumatic. *Atraumatics* are those in which the needle and thread have been commercially bonded together. When used for sewing, they create a continuous, small-diameter track through the tissues. As their name suggests, they cause minimal trauma.

Traumatics are needles and thread which are not attached. These needles have eyes, which need to be threaded with a length of suture material. As their name suggests, they cause relatively more trauma when used for sewing. A larger hole is made in the tissues, as the eye of the needle and a loop of thread have to be accommodated. As you can imagine, with the advent of atraumatics, traumatics are no longer in common use. You may see older surgeons use them from time to time; gynaecologists in particular seem to like them.

Let us now turn our attention back to the materials of which sutures are made. The following list is not exhaustive, but includes those in most common use. All sutures are made of materials foreign to the body, and therefore are all equally attacked by body enzymes. As a result, some are absorbed and some are not.

Absorbable sutures

These are used for suturing tissues which heal more rapidly and more satisfactorily; tissues which therefore only require temporary support until natural healing occurs. Some are made from mammal collagen fibres and some are synthetic.

The most commonly used absorbable suture is catgut, made from sheeps' intestines – nothing to do with cats! Catgut comes in two forms: plain and chromic catgut.

Plain catgut

As its name suggests, this is catgut in the raw state, untreated by any chemicals. It is therefore absorbed by the tissues more rapidly, usually within 5–10 days. It is commonly used for suturing subcutaneous tissue. Plain catgut is light tan in colour, and it is very springy material. It is best stretched before use and should be kept moist so that it does not become brittle.

Chromic catgut

This is catgut treated with a chromium salt solution, which renders it more resistant to digestion by the body's enzymes. It takes 10–20 days for absorption to occur, therefore it gives prolonged tissue support. It is commonly used to suture peritoneum and muscle fascia. It is distinguishable from plain catgut by its dark brown colouring, but should be handled in the same manner. As well as prolonged tissue support, it has another advantage over plain catgut – it is less irritant to the tissues and can be used in the presence of infection.

Dexon (polyglycolic acid)

This is a synthetic absorbable suture, which has been available since the early 1970s. It is green or white in colour, and takes about 12 weeks to be absorbed. It can be used for suturing all tissues, although it is not normally used on gut. It is stronger than catgut and more easily handled.

Vicryl (polyglactin 910)

This is a newer synthetic absorbable suture, available since the early 1980s. It is violet in colour, with an absorption rate of 10–12 weeks. Like dexon it is easy to handle, and can be used for suturing all tissues, including gut, where it is commonly used for anastomoses.

Non-absorbable sutures

These are sutures which are resistant to digestion by the body's enzymes. They are used to give permanent support to a wound, even after the natural healing process has occurred. As with absorbable sutures, some of these materials are natural and some synthetic.

Ethilon (nylon)

This is probably the most common non-absorbable suture in use. It is a synthetic material and is black, green or blue. It has a very elastic, springy texture, which requires extra knotting to prevent it from slipping. Ethilon has a good *tensile strength* – it can be put under a great deal of stress before it will break. It is commonly used for suturing abdominal muscle. It is also used on skin, from which it needs to be removed once the wound has healed.

Prolene

This is a similar synthetic material. It is blue in colour and its uses are similar to those of ethilon. It does have a few advantages however; it is less irritant to the tissues and can be used in the presence of infection, and it holds knots better. Very fine prolene sutures are widely used for anastomosing blood vessels.

Ethibond

This is a similar synthetic product. It is white or green and is commonly used for anastomosing blood vessels in cardiovascular surgery, and for anastomosing bowel in general surgery.

Silk

This is a natural non-absorbable material, composed of the fibres spun by silkworm larvae when making their cocoon. It is black and easy to handle. It can be used in most bodily tissues, but is less common today, making way for the stronger synthetic alternatives.

Linen

This is another natural material, made from flax. It is white in colour, and again easy to handle. It is commonly used for suturing gut and for tying off deep blood vessels.

Two commonly used terms relating to the composition of suture materials are monofilament and multifilament. *Monofilament* simply means that the suture is composed of a single strand of material. Common monofilaments are catgut, ethilon and prolene. *Multifilaments* are sutures composed of two or more strands of material, either twisted or braided together. Common multifilaments are dexon, vicryl, ethibond, silk and linen.

Suture gauges

Suture materials are available in different sized diameters, which are denoted by the suture's gauge. The thickest diameter available is a size 2, and they go down in thickness thus: 2, 1, 0, 2/0, 3/0, 4/0 etc. The finest diameter suture material available is a 10/0, which is so fine that it is difficult to see. This would be used for delicate nerve surgery. For general surgery, nothing much smaller than a 4/0 suture is used. Sizes 2 and 1 are used in coarser tissues, where plenty of tensile strength is needed, such as in suturing abdominal or back muscles. Sizes 0 and 2/0 are used for peritoneum, gut and subcutaneous tissue. Sizes 3/0 and 4/0 are suitable for use on skin, where a good cosmetic effect can be achieved, and for suturing smaller structures such as the common bile duct, the bladder and kidneys and for bowel anastomoses.

The finer range of sutures, sizes 4/0–10/0, are used in ophthalmics, blood vessel anastomoses and neurosurgery. (The metric sizes of suture diameters are also given on the packaging, adjacent to the gauge size, but these are almost never referred to in common use.)

Handling sutures is the only way to get to know them. All this information about tensile strength, springiness and the relative gauge sizes doesn't mean much when discussed in an abstract way. At the end of an operation, ask if you can look at any spare sutures, or those opened in error. (Do not touch any that have been used for suturing as you are at risk of contaminating yourself.) It is wasteful to open a new, sterile suture, as they can be very expensive. A chromic catgut suture costs 86p (in 1989) whereas something like a 10/0 nylon ophthalmic suture costs £9.42p.

NEEDLES

Needles vary in four respects: shape, length, heaviness and point.

Shape and length

These two features are governed by the same consideration. In general, needles are either straight or curved. *Straight needles* are used to suture subcutaneous tissue and skin and for securing wound drains. They can only be used at a superficial level, as manoeuvring them inside a wound would be impossible as it would cause unnecessary trauma to adjacent tissue.

Sewing at deeper levels requires a curved needle, as to suture here requires a semi-circular movement of the wrist, at the end of which the needle point must be facing upwards instead of puncturing adjacent tissue. (This is probably difficult to visualize, so when you are handling any spare sutures, imagine manoeuvring them in wounds of different depths. Better still, practise on a spare piece of foam rubber, in which you can cut your own wound.)

The amount of curve in each needle and its length vary according to the job for which the needle is designed and the amount of space available in which to do it. For example, a deep tension suture, used for supporting a weak abdominal wound, needs to be long to create a wide area of support around the wound and only needs a shallow curve, as it goes no deeper than the muscle layer. For sewing together two ends of bowel, the needle must be shorter and more fully curved in order to make neater, smaller movements. Thus needles can be straight, slightly curved, semi-circular or even more fully curved. They also vary in length, according to the extent of tissue 'bite' they are required to make.

Heaviness

The heaviness of a needle will always be in proportion to the gauge of suture material in atraumatic sutures. It makes sense that if you are going to suture a facial wound with 4/0 thread, then you need a fine needle. In fact the needles and thread are of exactly the same diameter, so there is no need to worry about matching the two up. When you choose a 2 or 1 gauge thread for suturing muscle, you can be sure that it will be attached to a thick, heavy needle appropriate for the job. Similarly, if you pick out a 2/0 or 3/0 thread, a finer, lighter needle will be attached. Needles, like suture material, vary in heaviness according to the coarseness of the tissue they are required to suture.

Points

Needle points fall roughly into two categories: cutting and round-bodied. *Cutting needles* are for suturing tough, coarse tissue, such as muscle and skin. Without a cutting edge it would be difficult to push a needle through. *Round-bodied needles* have a point, but no cutting edge. They are used for more delicate tissues, such as bowel or peritoneum, where a cutting edge would cause unnecessary trauma.

There is much variety in the shapes and sizes of cutting edges available, with reverse cutting needles, extra cutting and even spatula-shaped ones; these are refinements which you will appreciate with more time and experience. For now it is best to grasp the essential difference between cutting and round-bodied needles.

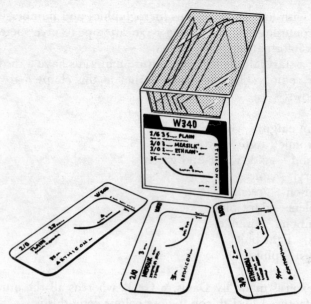

Fig. 7.1 Suture box and suture packets

SUTURE PACKAGING

All sutures are now commercially packed. They are double-wrapped with a peel-back, see-through outer wrapper, and an inner foil packet marked with all the suture details (Fig. 7.1). The foil packets have tear-down corners which when removed will expose the needle ready for mounting on a needleholder. The suture material is coiled around an inner piece of card. All sutures are packed dry, except for catgut, which is suspended in a solution of alcohol and water to help maintain its pliability. (Open these packets over a rubbish bag or container so that instruments are not contaminated by the solution. This could result in tissue irritation. Also protect your eyes.) All suture packets are sterilized by gamma irradiation.

IDENTIFYING SUTURES

Finding a specific suture from the rack is initially a formidable task, and one which may cause you considerable anxiety if the suture is needed in a hurry. These rows of different coloured boxes with lots of mysterious hieroglyphics and numbers are all very confusing. The following is an attempt to give some order to this information.

For a start, all the different suture materials have a distinctive colour coding. The ones listed earlier in this chapter are coded as follows:

1 Plain catgut – yellow.
2 Chromic catgut – brown.
3 Dexon – gold, white and green.
4 Vicryl – violet.
5 Ethilon – green.
6 Prolene – dark blue.
7 Ethibond – orange.
8 Silk – light blue.
9 Linen – pink.

(Dexon is made by Davis & Geck, whereas all the others are manufactured by Ethicon, whose colour code this is.)

The boxes should be grouped according to colour in the suture rack, for ease of location. The name of the suture material is also printed across the top of the box.

What about gauge size? On the top row of the information written on the white area of the suture box, the gauge is to be found on the right hand side, in brackets.

Now what about the needle? There should be a picture of the needle on the box. If there is no picture then there is no needle; you are looking at a box of ties. Inside the needle illustration is written the length of the needle in millimetres and the picture itself demonstrates how heavy the needle is. If two needles are pictured, then there are two in the pack, meaning that the suture is double-ended, i.e. it has a needle on both ends. Finally, above the needle is a symbol indicating what type of point it has. This is also written underneath. The two important symbols to recognize are:

● Round-bodied.

▲ Cutting needle Variations are:

◬ Trocar point (a cutting head that merges into a round body).

⊕   Tapercut.

▼   Reverse cutting.

◣   Spatulated needle.

Numbers

By now you are probably wondering where the suture numbers, on the top right hand corner of the box, fit in, such as 441, 788 etc. Their purpose is for ease of ordering, but you may find that the trained staff in your department ask for sutures by their number. They have been deliberately omitted so far, as using numbers is not helpful for learning about sutures and their use. It is much better if the scrub nurse asks you for a 2/0 chromic catgut suture on a round-bodied needle for the appendix stump, rather than for a 441. That way you learn much more quickly what is needed for the job, rather than searching for a number which masks all the other details. Knowing numbers is only useful if that number is in stock. What if it isn't? How will you improvise and find a similar one, since you have no idea what the suture behind the number is really like? What if you are not working with Ethicon sutures? If you choose a career in theatre nursing and work abroad, or even in a hospital in Britain which buys another brand of suture, then your learned numbers will be meaningless.

If numbers are always used in your department, get the scrub nurse to tell you at least what type of material the number refers to; this will cut down your searching time. When you have a quiet moment, study the other details on the pack.

HANDLING TIES AND SUTURES

Ties

Silk and linen ties come in lengths ready cut for use. You will have to cut dexon, vicryl and catgut yourself, usually into third lengths. Once cut, it is best to store them inside a folded small green towel, with both cut ends sticking out. This enables you to pull them out singly with ease and helps prevent them from becoming tangled. The silk and linen ties are secured together with a foil tag. This can be clipped on to a Mayo table, and again the ties can be removed singly with ease.

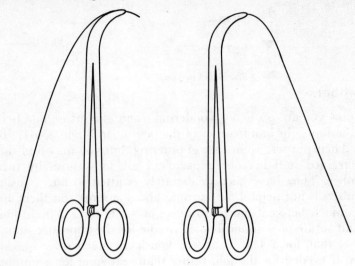

Fig. 7.2   Mounting ties

Remember that due to its springiness, the catgut will need to be stretched and to keep it from brittleness, it needs to be kept moist. So if your ties have been cut ready a long time before being used, dip them into some water before handing them to the surgeon.

To hand a tie, offer it stretched out at both ends, so that the surgeon can grasp it in the middle. For deep work, the tie will need to be mounted on to artery forceps, so that it can be passed with ease around the bleeding vessel (Fig. 7.2).

Sutures

When the tear-down corner of the inner foil packet is removed, the needle of the suture is ready and adequately exposed for mounting on a needleholder. As with instruments, avoid handling the needles more than is necessary. The needleholder is applied at right angles to the curve of the needle, just before the half-way point of the curve, towards the thread end. Application at this point allows space to manoeuvre the curve of the needle through the tissues. Try some other positions, and you will find that if you mount the needleholder too close to the thread end, you will not have such good control of the needle. If you mount it closer to the point of the needle, suturing becomes impossible. Before closing its ratchet, check that the needle is also mounted right at the tips of the needleholder. If it is mounted lower down, the needle is not well supported and will wobble. Try this as well.

Needles form part of your safety count, so always make sure that every needle is handed back to you after use, and is retained for counting. Some kind of adhesive pad for storing needles is useful, or else some scrub nurses thread them back through their original foil packets and store them in a receiver. Retaining the foil packets is a good extra safety check, as that way you are in no doubt as to how many needles you had throughout the course of the operation.

COMMON METHODS OF SUTURING

Continuous

As its name suggests, this is one long 'over and over' stitch, where only the first and last stitches are tied.

Interrupted

As its name suggests, this is where each stitch is tied separately. This facilitates removal of one or more stitches without disturbing the whole wound.

Subcuticular

This is a very neat way of closing a wound. It is a continuous stitch applied to subcutaneous tissue, in such a way as to approximate the skin edges, but avoiding actual stitch scars on the skin. The suture is knotted at either end and pulled tight. It is mainly used in gynaecological surgery, where it gives an excellent cosmetic effect.

Purse-string

This, as you might imagine, is a draw-string suture applied to a stump which is to be sealed off. The thread is stitched in and out of the edges of the stump, pulled tight, secured, and then the end of the stump is buried or invaginated. This stitch is most commonly used to seal off the appendix stump.

OTHER METHODS OF WOUND CLOSURE

Metal clips

These can be used to perform many of the functions of sutures, but are less common as a skin closure these days. The teeth of the clips tend to leave ugly scars, but they do have the advantage of much quicker removal. This explains why they are still always used in thyroid surgery, where it is essential to be able to open the wound swiftly should haemorrhage occur. *Kifa and Michel clips* are the two types of clips most commonly used in skin closure.

Ligaclips are finer, less traumatic metal clips, which can be used like ligatures. They can be applied to deep bleeding vessels, or to nerve fibres, as in a lumbar sympathectomy.

There is definite growth in the use of metal clips in one area however, and that is in anastomosis formation in the alimentary tract. The clips used here are ready-packed in sterile cartridges for application with a surgical gun. These clips are very expensive, but this is countered by the fact that the surgeon can perform neat, quick operations with them.

Steristrips

These also have a place in skin closure. They can be used in addition to a subcuticular stitch, to give gentle support to the skin edges, or else in conjunction with skin sutures on wounds where it is difficult to get a good approximation.

DRESSINGS

Now that the wound has been effectively closed, cleaned and dried, it needs to be dressed. The main objectives in dressing a wound are firstly to cover it, in such a way as to promote healing by maintaining a moist, contamination-free environment where gaseous exchange across the dressing is uninhibited, and secondly to immobilize it. Movement leads to pain and slower healing. Above all, the patient should find the dressing as comfortable as possible, allowing as much freedom of movement to the rest of the body as possible; the dressing should also be made of a material which is not an irritant. The following are some general guidelines to the kinds of dressings you will meet in the operating department.

Large wounds

Be they abdominal or orthopaedic, these wounds are normally covered with large waterproof strip dressings, such as Airstrip or Mepore, the non-irritant version. These dressings have three layers: a non-stick layer directly over the wound, an absorbent layer to hold any exudate, and an outer protective, sealing layer. Alternatively, transparent dressings of the Opsite variety may be used. These promote good wound healing and have the added advantage of allowing wound inspection without the need to disturb the dressing.

If *wound drains* are present, these are normally dressed separately for ease of inspection and changing and to prevent contamination of the main wound. Drains are invariably dressed with gauze squares with a cut-out keyhole or slit to fit snugly around the drain. This is supported by light strapping such as Micropore.

Smaller wounds

These can also be dressed with a waterproof strip, but where there is likely to be less exudate and more rapid healing, gauze squares and light strapping will be sufficient. Alternatively, a spray dressing can be used, which acts as an extra layer of skin. In this way the wound is covered by a transparent semi-permeable membrane, through which oxygen can pass and promote more rapid healing.

Extra support

This will need to be added to dressings over sites where oedema or haematoma is more likely to occur. This support can be given by adding a layer of padding over gauze squares, usually with cotton wool or a dressing pad. If the wound is on a limb, this will need to be supported by a crêpe bandage. If on the torso, elastocrêpe is better. Most *orthopaedic wounds* are dressed in this manner. Other examples where extra support is needed are following breast lump biopsy or stripping and ligation of varicose veins.

Remember to use the correct size of *crêpe bandage*: 6″ are used for legs, 4″ for arms and head dressings, while 2″ are suitable for toes, feet, fingers and hands. Tougher strapping is needed to secure the bandages, such as zinc oxide.

Raw areas

Where the top layer of skin is absent, such as over the toenail bed after the removal of an ingrowing nail, or over a skin graft donor site, such raw areas need an extra protective layer beneath the gauze. This is necessary to prevent the gauze from sticking, which will not only have a detrimental effect upon healing, but will cause excruciating pain when it is removed. A layer of paraffin gauze usually fits the bill.

Cavities

Cavities likely to bleed postoperatively are usually packed with a gauze roll to apply pressure to the bleeding points, for example in the vagina following vaginal hysterectomy.

Artificially created cavities which need to heal, such as those left after incision and drainage of an abscess, are also usually packed with ribbon gauze to allow wick drainage.

If a *plaster of Paris* cast is to be applied to a limb, a protective layer of orthopaedic wool must be applied over the dressing. This is less bulky than ordinary cotton wool. It is presented in the form of a bandage, so the same sizing as for crêpe bandages applies.

WOUND DRAINAGE SYSTEMS

Wounds are drained for two reasons: firstly, to prevent haematoma formation, and secondly, as a temporary diversion for other body fluids while healing occurs. Collection of any of these fluids – such as bile, urine or pus – in the tissues would seriously interfere with the process.

Draining blood

This is normally done by means of a suction or vacuum drain. These are introduced at a point away from the main wound, and stitched in place. They consist of a metal introducer which screws into the perforated drainage tube, a length of connecting tubing, and finally the graduated bottle with a vacuum seal. (The metal introducers are very sharp and should be handled with care. Once the drain is in position, the introducers can be cut off and disposed of in the same way that needles and blades are dealt with; unless of course your hospital recycles them.) Once the wound is closed the vacuum clamp on the bottle can be released, and blood will normally be seen tracking down the tubing immediately. These drains are normally removed 48 hours postoperatively.

Chest drains

These drains have two purposes. They can be used to re-inflate a collapsed lung or to drain any fluid collection between the pleura following thoracic surgery. They work by maintaining a negative pressure within the chest, which is necessary for normal respiration to occur.

The plastic drainage tube and the connecting tubing are similar to those of other suction drains, but with a much larger bore. It is the bottles which are very different. They are tall and cylindrical, with measuring gradations and a much larger capacity. Before use they must be filled with 200 ml of sterile water. (This level must be clearly marked, so that drainage can be accurately estimated.) They have a rubber bung at the top, through which two plastic tubes pass. One is much longer than the other, and it is this one which connects to the drainge tubing from the chest. Its distal end will be below the water level so that an underwater seal is created (Fig. 7.3). Following thoracic surgery, drainage is controlled naturally by the patient's respiratory rate. Fluid is expelled during expiration and flows downwards into the drainage bottle, as it is heavier than air. On inspiration a little water is drawn back up the drainage tubing, but do not worry, this cannot harm the patient. The tubing is too long and the water too heavy for it to travel very far. It certainly will not get as far as the chest.

Chest drains are therefore not suction drains. A pre-set suction pressure would interfere with respiration, and suction drainage bottles could not cope with the often very large volumes of exudate from the chest. Suction drainage bottles can sometimes lose their vacuum too, whereas provided that all the chest drain connections are secure, the water gives a constant seal. This is an important point, as obviously it is a serious matter if the seal is lost. The condition of the patient will deteriorate immediately as the lung collapses. Clearly it is of the greatest importance always

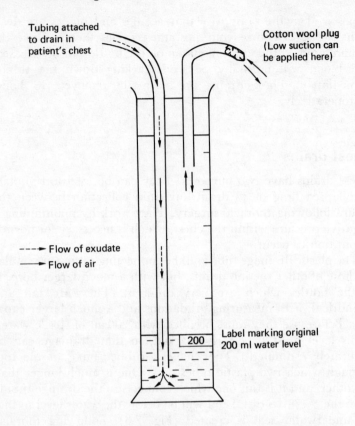

Tubing attached
to drain in
patient's chest

Cotton wool plug
(Low suction can
be applied here)

---→ Flow of exudate
——→ Flow of air

200　Label marking original
200 ml water level

Fig. 7.3　Chest drain and how it works

to ensure sound connections. (Sleek strapping is often applied at these points for greater safety.) Although chest drains are not suction drains, electrical low suction machines can be applied to the shorter tubing emerging from the rubber bung, to increase the negative pressure within the chest.

Two strong Spencer Wells clamps must always be at hand to clamp the tubing if alterations need to be made to the bung or if the bottle needs emptying. Without the clamps, air would be sucked into the chest, resulting in pneumothorax. The clamps must also be used when lifting or moving the patient. If the bottles were lifted to the level of the patient's chest or above without the clamps in situ, water would siphon into the chest.

Other fluids

More viscous fluids, such as *pus*, are drained by soft rubber or plastic tissue drains, such as Yeats, corrugated, Ragnell or Paul's tubing. These are not normally sutured in place, but instead are secured with a large safety pin through the protruding end to stop them slipping back into the wound. They are covered with gauze at the end of operation. As the exudate lessens, the drains are gradually shortened to allow the tract to heal from below, until they are finally removed several days postoperatively.

T-tubes are a distinctive type of soft plastic tubing, used to drain the common *bile* duct after stones have been removed. As their name suggests, they are T-shaped. The cross of the T sits in the common bile duct, while the long stem is brought out through the skin and attached to a graduated drainage bag. Again this is gradually shortened, spigoted, and finally removed when the surgeon is happy that bile is draining normally into the duodenum.

Urine

This has to be drained with a much larger-bore rigid type of tubing, as it is much less concentrated and produced by the body in much larger volumes. The drains are perforated and attach to a normal urine bag. These drains need to be stitched in place.

Further reading

Ethicon Inc. (1977). *Suture Use Manual: Use and Handling of Sutures and Needles*, 3rd ed. Edinburgh: Ethicon.
Moody, M. (ed.) (1988). Tissue viability, wound care. *Nursing Times/Nursing Mirror*, **84**(2), pp. 62–70.
Scott, M. (1983). 32,000 years of sutures. *NAT News*, **20**(5), pp. 15–17.

8

The role of the circulating nurse

This will be your first role in the operating theatre before you are ready to scrub up for cases. In fact that's not quite true; what you are most likely to be doing initially is observing the role of the circulator, and participating as and when you feel able. For the role of the circulator is a complex one, and although the scrub nurse role appears more glamorous and at the same time daunting, most theatre nurses would agree that circulating is more demanding. To function in the role intelligently demands forethought and a wealth of knowledge of surgery and the department. These skills are aquired in time. For the present, we will break down the role of the circulating nurse, and look at some of the specific activities with which you will be expected to help.

Firstly, all the major concerns of the role should be identified. What thoughts colour the circulating nurse's judgements? What are his or her priorities? There are three major concerns. Firstly, care of the patient's safety and that of the staff. Second, the maintenance of asepsis; thirdly, allegiance to the scrub nurse. The role involves working very closely with the scrub nurse and being constantly alert to his or her needs in particular. The scrub nurse must *never* be left without a circulator.

ORIENTATION

To function as a circulating nurse, you must first of all familiarize yourself with the geography of the suite and the department. Outside the suite, you will need to know where the nearest defibrillator is, the nearest telephone, and fire appliances and exits. In time you will also need to find all the stockrooms; where to get extra instruments, blades, sutures, dressings, disposal bags and stationery.

evaporate.) Like the gowns, trays of instruments are also double-wrapped; check for sterility in the same manner. The outer wrapper is normally removed in the theatre corridor, as it is considered to be the dust cover. The tray is transferred on to the clean trolley with the inner wrapper exposed. This layer is not opened until the trolley is inside the clean preparation room. The trays are much larger than gown packs and so are the risks of you contaminating them if you lean across them to open the inner wrap. Walk around the trolley as you open the different sides; remember to observe the invisible barrier! If there are instruments in the autoclave to be used, you can open the door ready for the scrub nurse once the cycle is complete.

Opening extras

Once the scrub nurse has arranged the instruments, there will be packs of sutures, ties, swabs, blades and other extras which he or she will need you to open. The speed of this procedure must be dictated by the scrub nurse. Never harass him or her by dropping lots of things on to the trolley when he or she is not ready for them. Instead, let the scrub nurse take things from you individually, at his or her own pace, double-checking each piece.

Sutures, ties, blades and the majority of commercially packed items come in peel-back wrappers. Standing well back behind the invisible barrier around the trolley, peel these open, and offer the contents to the scrub nurse, who will take the items with a pair of long handling forceps. Hospital packed equipment will probably be wrapped in double paper bags. Check these for sterility, break the autoclave tape seal, and open the outer bag by sliding your fingers up the side gussets. There is no need to touch the folded-over top of the bag; this will open automatically as you move your fingers. It is through the top of the bag that the scrub nurse must put sterile forceps, or else occasionally a gloved hand if the contents of the bag are heavy.

Checking lotions

Skin preparation lotion will also be needed. Show the label on the bottle to the scrub nurse, so that you can both verify the correct solution and check the expiry date. Then break the sterile seal on the bottle, and with your hand over the label (to preserve its legibility), pour the lotion into the offered container from a height of at least 15 cm. Remember that while the contents of the bottle are sterile, the outside of the bottle is not! Many solutions are now widely available in commercially prepared sachets. These should be checked in the same manner, with the awareness that different companies call the same solutions by different names – their own trade names. Take extra care and be sure that you both agree that you have the correct solution. The sachets are opened by tearing off the corner marked by the manufacturer, and again, pouring from a height.

Drugs

If any other drugs are required on the scrub nurse's trolley, such as an ampoule of local anaesthetic, you must check the drug and the expiry date with the surgeon as well as the scrub nurse before it is drawn up for use. Unless the ampoule has been specially prepared in a sterile pack, break off the top, using a piece of green gauze to protect your fingers, and offer it to the scrub nurse so that he or she can insert a needle or filling tube.

PERFORMING THE FIRST COUNT

Before the operation commences, the number of instruments, swabs and needles on the trolley must be counted and recorded. The purpose of this is to ensure that none of these items are left inside the patient at the end of operation. Everything is counted again at the end, so the scrub nurse and surgeon can be sure that everything that was on the trolley originally, still is. The counting is done by two nurses, one of whom is the scrub nurse, and one of the two must be qualified. Most hospitals have a special count sheet for recording this information, or else it may be written up on a board inside the theatre.

To check the instruments, use the check sheet from the pre-packed tray, and call out the contents, which the scrub nurse must show you. Any instruments added to the basic tray must be recorded on the count sheet. To check the number of needles, count together the number of needle symbols on the suture packs. Hypodermic and any other types of needles should also be counted, and their number written in a separate space on the count sheet.

When checking swabs, you are counting the number present

and also checking that each swab has an individual safety marker. Swabs have historically been the items most commonly left inside patients, so now they all have a black Raytec strip woven into them, which is x-ray detectable. Then if there is any discrepancy in the final count, as a last resort the patient can be x-rayed on the operating table to determine whether or not there is a swab still in the wound. Large swabs also have tapes attached as an extra safeguard. These can be left hanging outside the wound as a reminder that the swab is in there. Small artery forceps can be attached to the tapes to draw extra attention to them. So, when counting, the scrub nurse will remove the tie around the bundle of swabs, and you will count together out loud that five are present and that all five are safety-marked or taped as appropriate. (All swabs are packed in bundles of five. Any packs containing a different number should be discarded immediately, as this would render the count very confusing.) Record each five after counting, entering the different sizes of swabs in the appropriate columns on the count sheet.

Other items which could easily be lost, such as slings, nylon tapes and gauze rolls (also with a Raytec marker) are counted and recorded on the sheet too (Fig. 8.1).

It cannot be over-emphasized that the count sheet is very important and must be filled in correctly. Counting accurately is also important. Make sure that you really do count together out loud and that you actually see each item. If you are at all uncertain, ask the scrub nurse to repeat the count. You must be entirely happy, as you are required to sign the count sheet – a legal document – stating that the count is accurate. Make sure that yours and the scrub nurses's names are also entered correctly. The count sheet then goes into the theatre where a running record of swabs, instruments and needles is kept on it throughout the operation. It will soon become second nature to you to record any additions.

PATIENT SAFETY

Before the operation begins, you must turn your attention to the safety of the patient, who will by now be inside the theatre, anaesthetized on the operating table. If any alteration to position is necessary, for example if he or she needs to be in the lithotomy position or a varicose veins board needs to be inserted before

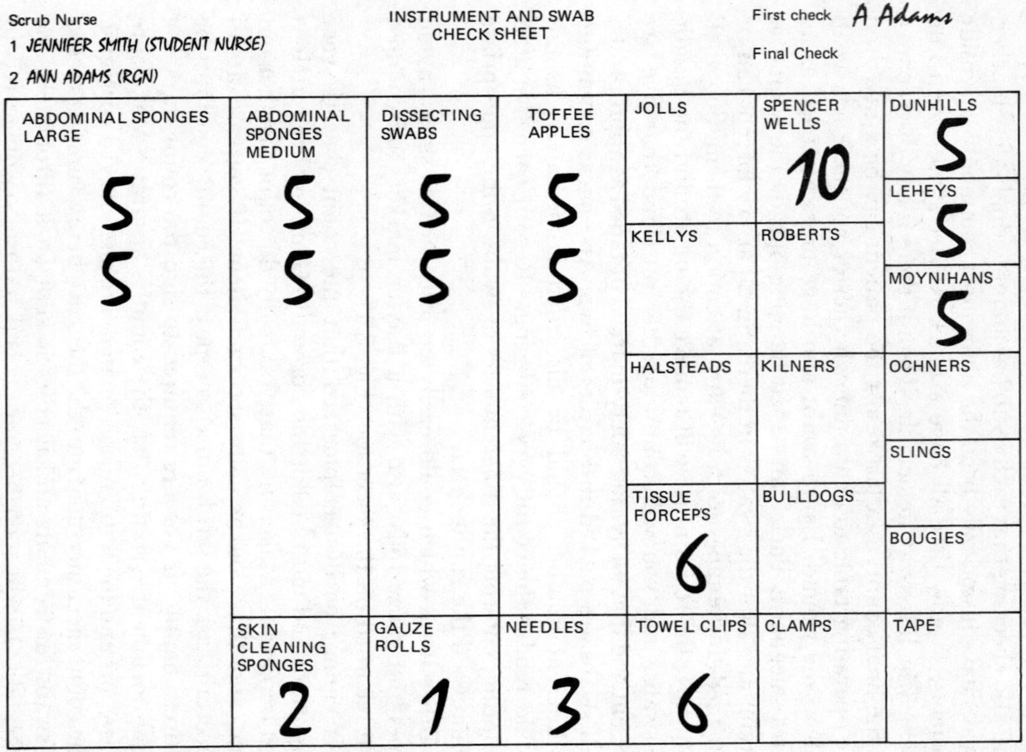

Scrub Nurse
1 JENNIFER SMITH (STUDENT NURSE)
2 ANN ADAMS (RGN)

INSTRUMENT AND SWAB CHECK SHEET

First check A Adams
Final Check

ABDOMINAL SPONGES LARGE	ABDOMINAL SPONGES MEDIUM	DISSECTING SWABS	TOFFEE APPLES	JOLLS	SPENCER WELLS	DUNHILLS
5 5	5 5	5 5	5 5		10	5
						LEHEYS 5
				KELLYS	ROBERTS	MOYNIHANS 5
				HALSTEADS	KILNERS	OCHNERS
						SLINGS
				TISSUE FORCEPS 6	BULLDOGS	BOUGIES
	SKIN CLEANING SPONGES 2	GAUZE ROLLS 1	NEEDLES 3	TOWEL CLIPS 6	CLAMPS	TAPE

Fig. 8.1 A completed count sheet

surgery is possible, remember to move the patient gently so as not to put undue strain on the limbs or joints. Now you must think to yourself, is the patient safe? Is he or she in danger of sustaining pressure sores? Check that all pressure points are adequately padded (see Chapter 2). Could he or she sustain a diathermy burn? Make sure that the diathermy plate is in position, with good contact with an area of dry skin, and that the plate lead is hanging freely, where it will not be covered up by the drapes. See that the patient is in contact with no other metal, such as drip stands, lithotomy poles or the diathermy machine itself, as burns could occur at these sites. Finally, is the patient in danger of sustaining any damage to nerves? Make sure that all limbs are securely positioned. A limb which hangs over the edge of the table during a long operation may suffer irreparable damage.

These safety checks must be done before the green drapes go on, and done properly. If not, any omissions will not be discovered until after the operation is over, when it is too late to remedy the situation.

Think also of the patient's dignity. The gown does not need to be tucked away from the site of operation until the surgeon is just about to clean the skin. At this point, you can quickly check to see that the area has been adequately shaved by the ward staff. (Obviously it is undesirable to shave in the theatre, as loose hairs left on the surface could contaminate the wound. If it is necessary, be sure to remove the hair with some wide Elastoplast strapping.) Any existing dressings or ostomy appliances will need to be removed. Put disposable gloves on to do this and have a disposal bag ready. This bag may be removed from the theatre now as the operation has not started. Once it does, *nothing leaves the theatre*. The reason for this is to ensure the accuracy of the count. If there is a discrepancy, all the disposal bags have to be checked for the missing item (see below). You can now switch on the operating lights and position them over the wound site.

ARRANGING FURNITURE

While the surgeon is cleaning the skin, you can help the scrub nurse to arrange the trolleys comfortably. Until the scrub nurse is settled, do not move any other equipment, such as the diathermy or suction machine, into position. This just creates more hazards to negotiate; moving trolleys over electrical leads, and putting them at greater risk of desterilization. When the surgeon has finished cleaning, he or she will hand out to you the container of lotion and the cleaning sponges. (Take care not to contaminate the surgeon's gloves.) Place these on the bottom shelf of the swab rack where they can easily be located when closing counts are performed.

Once the sterile green drapes are on, you can move the necessary equipment closer to the patient. If a Mayo table is to be used, move this in over the patient's feet first, as the scrub nurse can then get on and lay out the instruments ready to commence surgery. Next, the diathermy machine: this is usually best at the foot of the table. Plug in the patient lead, and ensure that the machine is switched on at the mains. Connect the sterile diathermy lead handed out to you, and switch the diathermy on. Check which coagulation or cutting setting the surgeon wishes to use, and call this out as you set the dial. It is best to confirm any setting changes in this way. Finally, check that the surgeon has the appropriate foot pedals. (If he or she changes position during the operation, remember to move the pedals as well.) With both the Mayo table and the diathermy machine, make sure that the patient's feet are free of contact, which could lead to pressure sores or diathermy burns. Connect the suction tubing and switch the suction on. Any other leads needed for the operation, such as fibreoptic light leads or compressed air leads, should also be connected to their light sources or cylinders as appropriate at this point.

Once the furniture is all in place, and surgery has commenced, take a cool, logical look at everything, to see if things can be improved. Does the scrub nurse have a swab disposal bowl within reach? Can he or she see the swab rack? Are all the trolleys and bowl stands within easy reach? All this furniture is on wheels. Has sterile water been put into the bowls, and has the surgeon got a 'splash' bowl? To be a good circulating nurse you need empathy – the ability to imagine yourself in the shoes of others, recognizing their needs before being asked. Also ask yourself, is the environment safe? Is there any furniture on which the scrub team are likely to desterilize themselves if they turn round quickly? Are there any leads which might trip people up? If these cannot be rearranged more safely, it is a good idea to adhere the leads to the floor with sleek strapping. Is anyone in danger of banging their head on the operating light? If there is no easy way to avoid these hazards, you can at least ask the scrub nurse to warn the members of the team at risk. Having a comfortable scrub team minimizes frustration and stress and benefits everyone, not least the patient, who has a quicker, smoother operation.

Now that both patient and staff are safe and comfortable, check again that you have at hand more swabs, blades, sutures and any additional items collected by the scrub nurse. Make sure you have the count sheet at the ready to add anything.

From now on, the role of the circulating nurse is largely being alert and responding to the needs of the scrub team. This involves seeing that all the equipment in use functions as it should. For example, changing the position of the operating lights as necessary, noticing if new air cylinders or infusion bags are needed, observing suction bottles to see if they need changing or emptying and observing urine drainage too. In the latter two cases the anaesthetist usually likes to know the amount of blood or urine discarded, which should be added to running totals on the swab board. You need to notice how much sterile equipment is being used and take steps to remedy the situation if stocks are being depleted. While the scrub team are engrossed in the operation, the circulator ensures the smooth running of the environment and back-up services. There are several other specific activities which constitute such support; these are described below.

WEIGHING AND HANGING SWABS

During the operation, the scrub nurse will discard soaked swabs into a bowl on the floor. As all swabs must be accounted for, it is the circulator's job to hang them up on the swab rack for counting before they can be transferred to the swab bin. A special watch must also be kept for any swabs accidentally dropped on the floor elsewhere around the table. As in the initial count, swabs are again hung in groups of five according to type. Different types are hung on separate shelves of the rack. Use spongeholding forceps or wear gloves when you handle swabs; never use bare hands, as there is always the risk of contracting blood-borne infections. Open the swabs out as much as possible to ensure that only one is present. Large swabs with tapes should be hung in such a way that the tapes are clearly visible for counting. When you have collected five of one type, find a convenient moment to count them out loud with the scrub nurse. These can then be discarded into the swab bin, and you must straight away cross off five from the count sheet.

All swabs remain in the theatre until the end of the operation. Even if a second disposal bag has to be used to cope with a large volume of swabs, the first must remain in the theatre. The reason for this is that if there is a discrepancy in the closing counts, it may be necessary to recount the discarded swabs. If the first bag was taken out to the sluice during the operation, it would become mixed up with the bags of discarded swabs from previous operations, and then you could never distinguish the bag needed for recall. This means that you could never be 100 per cent certain that the swab count for the operation was accurate, and the patient would be needlessly subjected to yet another x-ray.

HUNTING FOR LOST SWABS

If a swab is missing during the closing counts, and you have searched fruitlessly for it in every conceivable hiding place – on the floor, under the table, in the specimen dish (common during caesarean sections) and in the surgeon's boots – then the next step is to recount discarded swabs. This is a messy procedure, so lay some sheets of waterproof paper on the floor before tipping the used swabs out. Wearing gloves, or using forceps, lay the swabs out in groups of five again, and again count them together with the scrub nurse. If the swab is still missing, you must continue to search in the other disposal bins – in the linen and rubbish bins. Again, carefully empty the contents on to some waterproof paper and sift through them. Hopefully by now the swab will have turned up. If not, and the scrub nurse has again searched through the drapes, on the trolley and in the rubbish bag, the patient must be x-rayed as a final resort. After all, everyone's prime concern is not to count for the love of it, but to be sure that the swab has not been left inside the patient, where it will initiate a postoperative infection. The same procedure is followed for lost instruments, needles, slings etc.; again remember that nothing leaves the theatre once the operation is underway.

As mentioned in Chapter 2, swabs are not weighed during every operation, but in those where the blood loss is expected to be of a degree to warrant replacement by the anaesthetist. The weight of the swabs tells him or her how much to replace. Swabs are normally weighed during major surgery and during operations on neonates. If in doubt, ask the anaesthetist. Large swabs are weighed singly before being hung on the rack, but it is best to weigh small ones in groups of fives for greater accuracy (see Chapter 2 for details of how to calculate blood loss). Remember to keep the running total of blood loss up-to-date on the swab board.

The swab rack is also a good place to display dropped or discarded instruments or needles. Using the bottom shelf or a row of spare hooks, the items can be grouped according to type where they are clearly visible to the scrub nurse. Again this facilitates counting. If something is accidentally dropped from the table, pick it up straight away and show it to the scrub nurse. He or she needs to know immediately what instrument is out of action. It may be that he or she will ask you for a replacement, or if this is not available, you will be asked to wash and resterilize the particular item.

HANDLING SPECIMENS

This is a very important aspect of the work of the circulating nurse, which must be done with care. Some operations are purely diagnostic, such as an excision biopsy of breast lump or a staging laparotomy. The specimens obtained are the purpose of the operation, and will determine the patient's diagnosis and subsequent management. So handle with great care!

When the scrub nurse hands you a specimen, there are several questions you need to ask. 'What is it? Where is it from? (Is it from the right hand side or the left? From the anterior or posterior wall?) What investigation does the surgeon require? (Histology, cytology, microbiology or something else?) Does the specimen need to be put into a preservative?' Choose an appropriate sized container for the specimen and label it clearly. On the label is written the patient's name, central registration number, ward, the name of the specimen and the date. Remember always to label the side of a container and not the lid. Once in the laboratory, the lid is the first thing to be removed, so there is always the danger of this vital information being lost.

Most specimens obtained at operation are for histology, and can be put into the preservative formol saline. The correct amount to use will just cover the specimen. Specimens for microbiology may be left dry or else put into a culture medium. These need to go to the laboratory as soon as possible, or else into a refrigerator if the laboratory is closed. Specimens for frozen section also remain dry and go immediately to the laboratory, where medical staff will have arranged for them to have priority investigation. Surgeons like some specimens to remain dry so that they can examine them after the operation before they finally go for histology. The gallbladder is one such case; the surgeon normally likes to dissect it after operation to see how many stones it contains.

All specimens must be accompanied by an appropriate request card, completed properly and signed by a member of the medical staff. (This is actually a medical staff responsibility, but it will benefit the patient if you can check this too.) There may also be a specimen register in the department, in which details of all the specimens sent must be entered. This helps to locate lost specimens.

Remember that specimens are a potential source of infection. You are exposed to this risk, along with the porters who deliver them to the laboratories, and the laboratory staff themselves. As soon as the specimen is correctly labelled it is best to put it into a plastic transporter bag to protect everyone else who comes into contact with it. In these days of increased awareness of the threat posed by blood-borne infections, it is now common practice to pack specimens in two layers of plastic transporter bags.

TAKING AND GIVING MESSAGES

One of the major functions of the circulating nurse is to act as a link between the scrubbed team and the outside world. Consequently, much of your time may be taken up with taking and giving messages. Obviously, if there are receptionists in your department, it is best if they answer telephones and bleeps, but this is not always possible. If the telephone outside your theatre rings, answer it as soon as you can. A ringing telephone is distracting and stressful.

If you do take a message, make sure you write down all the details accurately: the name of the person ringing, the time, the message, and a bleep or extension number where the caller can be contacted. It is best to take only one message, and to say that the person in question is scrubbed in theatre and will phone between operations, rather than getting involved in running to and fro, answering a string of queries. If you can, give some idea of how long the person being called will be occupied. Be wary of complicated messages or any that contain vital information which must be extremely accurate. You should certainly not get involved in repeating drug dosages over the telephone. If you are not happy to deliver a particular message, then say so. Answering the telephone takes you out of the theatre and away from helping the scrub nurse, which is a higher priority, so do not tarry long.

Having taken the message, you need to deliver it. It is not always easy to judge when to give a message, especially if the operation has just reached that delicate stage where absolute concentration is vital. It may be that the message is not so important that it needs to be known immediately, but can easily wait until the surgeon unscrubs. (Mr Jones will not thank you for bursting in and asking the houseman about Mrs Smith's sleeping tablets when he is in the process of dissecting an aneurysm!) Refer all messages to the trained staff and let them decide. If you are told that the message is very urgent, and the person on the line insists on waiting for an immediate answer, tell the message to the scrub nurse and let him or her deliver it. Leave any written messages in a safe place where the surgeons will find them, and remind them of their existence after the operation.

If you are given any messages regarding the details of patients on the operating list or any changes to the list itself, it is vital to tell the nurse in charge immediately. Indeed if you are not sure of the significance of any message you take, always relay it to the nurse in charge and let him or her decide.

CLOSING AND FINAL COUNTS

Once the surgeon begins to close the wound, the scrub nurse and circulating nurse need to count all the instruments, swabs and needles again. This is to ensure that nothing has been left at the site of operation. Normally two counts are done; one when the first cavity is closed, for example the uterus or peritoneum, and a final one as the skin is sutured. This is flexible however. More than two counts or perhaps only one can be done, depending on the scale of the operation and the wishes of the scrub nurse. The one criterion that must be satisfied is that at the end of operation, both the scrub nurse and circulating nurse are sure that nothing is missing.

The first count signals that the end of the operation is near. You can start to make preparations now for clearing the theatre, and more importantly, despatching the patient safely. Perhaps the suction can be switched off now and the bottles emptied. Are there any extra unused instruments that could be put away? Perhaps cylinders and light source machines can be disconnected and pushed to the side walls. Always ask first however, before removing any equipment. The patient's notes and x-rays can be gathered up and put ready for departure. You know that soon the skin will be closed, so ask what dressing will be required. You can put this out ready, along with any drainage bottles, strappings or skin cleaning lotions necessary. Gauze dressings are never opened before the final swab count. This is a safety measure to ensure that no gauze squares are mistaken for swabs when counting. This could render the count inaccurate and mask any discrepancy.

Once the final count has been done, and the scrub nurse is happy for you to do so, the swabs can be taken down from the rack and put into the swab bin. As there is little risk of bleeding now, the diathermy machine can be switched off, the patient lead unplugged and the machine pushed aside. (Leave the diathermy plate on the patient a while longer. Should any bleeding occur before the skin is closed, or indeed just after, the diathermy can swiftly be set up for use again.) You are clearing a safe space in which the patient can be lifted and transferred, and one in which the scrubbed team can move without danger of tripping over leads and banging into equipment. Remember to sign for any counts you have done.

BETWEEN CASES

Once the patient's wound has been dressed, the green drapes can be removed and placed in the linen bin. Before becoming involved in further clearing and cleaning of the theatre, remember that patient safety is your top priority. Is the patient safe and warm? Is he or she unnecessarily exposed? Arrange the operating gown in a dignified manner and remove the diathermy plate and any other equipment no longer necessary for monitoring or maintaining a safe position. If the patient is still intubated, and it seems as though it will be some time before he or she will be transferred back to the trolley, cover him or her up with a blanket to keep warm. (This is epecially important for small children and the elderly.) There must be one nurse constantly in attendance until the patient reaches recovery, to respond to the needs of both the patient and the anaesthetist.

As long as the patient's needs are catered for, you can help the scrubbed team out of their gowns and help the scrub nurse to wheel the trolleys out to the sluice. Remove the full disposal bags from the theatre, and leave them near the trolleys so that the scrub nurse can add his or her own linen and rubbish. Fresh bags need to be put out and some cleaning in the theatre is also necessary. The swab rack and swab bowls need wiping over with a damp cloth and some detergent solution, as do any other surfaces splashed with blood or other fluids. Remember to wear gloves! The floor may need some attention too, but take care when you mop it not to leave it too wet and slippery if there are more operations to follow. Clean, unsterile green towels can be used for drying surfaces. Even if there is another nurse in attendance, never be oblivious to what is happening to the patient as you go about the cleaning. Keep your eyes and ears open so that you too can respond if any help is needed. Usually it is a case of 'all hands on deck' when the patient needs to be lifted or turned. Care of the patient, as always, is top priority.

If this is the last patient on the list, more thorough cleaning of the theatre is necessary. All surfaces need damp dusting with detergent solution. Begin high up with the operating lights, and work downwards, removing dust and splashes of blood and other fluids as you go. The theatres are cleaned by commercial cleaners in the evenings. In particular, they give the floor a thorough wash by machine.

ANTICIPATION

The main components of the role of the circulating nurse have been listed here. With time, when you have observed the repetition of these activities, you will learn the normal sequence of events and be able to anticipate the next step. The ability to anticipate well is often cited as the cardinal virtue, if not the very essence of a good circulating nurse. It certainly is a bonus for everyone else, especially the scrub nurse, if the circulator can be relied on to be constantly alert and supply him or her with everything necessary before he or she has to break concentration to ask for it. Time is thus saved for everyone.

You may not think so, but even when you are new to theatre you can still anticipate some needs. If you see on the count sheet that the scrub nurse is down the last five swabs and the first closing count has not yet been done, the chances are that some more will be needed. So have another pack at the ready. You don't even need to ask if they are needed; these things are usually accomplished by a nod or a look from the scrub nurse. If you notice that the surgeon is using a lot of one particular suture, check that there is a good stock available in the theatre, and replenish them if not. If in its name the operation entails taking a specimen, such as excision biopsy of breast lump or dilatation and curettage, you can have the appropriate request card and suitable pot ready in advance. This is particularly helpful in a list with a fast turnover of short operations. (Do not label more than one pot in advance however, as mix-ups could occur.) When the closing count is performed, you know that a dressing will be required soon, so find the right one and have it to hand. If you see someone scrubbing up, check that a gown and gloves are open ready. It is a great help to everyone if you can be alert to their needs, and can supply some without having to be asked.

WATCHING AND LEARNING

So far we have only discussed learning through the performance of practical activities. This was deliberate, as it is not knowing what to do or how to do it which causes students most anxiety, coupled with the feeling that they are obliged to be constantly doing something. This is a pity. You will learn an awful lot if you can just relax and watch the surgery. Most of you feel unable to do this, fearing that others will think you lazy or slacking in your duties. If you are not the only circulating nurse, there is no reason why you should not ask at the beginning of the operation if you can simply watch, while they take care of the other responsibilities. Having established an agreement, you should be able to concentrate on watching and learning. If any questions occur to you, ask the trained staff to explain or to get the surgeon to explain to you. Make the most of the time when you are seeing how surgery is performed. If you are the only circulating nurse, obviously you cannot watch all the time, but make use of those periods when there is nothing immediate to be done.

For those of you still anxious about 'doing', there are always useful jobs to be done. Theatres consume an enormous amount of disposable equipment, as you will no doubt have noticed, so if you feel at a loose end, you can always make a stocking-up list. If there is another circulator, you may be able to leave the theatre to collect these items. Because of the number of personnel and the amount of activity in theatres, things get very untidy. Try to preserve an ordered environment. One area particularly affected is the scrup-up. This gets very messy; sinks and taps are splashed with soap solutions, the floor gets wet and brushes and paper towels are strewn about. A wet floor is a particular hazard to staff safety. This can be dried with clean, unsterile green towels.

There may be items not dealt with by the TSSU which need packing for sterilization. Have the trained staff teach you how to do this; which method of sterilization is to be used, and how to label the packs correctly. (This should not be done too close to the operating table, as the rustle of paper can be distracting.) If there is another operation to follow, you can help prepare the equipment as far as you are able, arranging clean trolleys and the appropriate trays or linen packs. The inner wrappers of trays should not be opened, however, until the next scrub nurse begins to scrub up.

These are some ideas for those of you who feel that you cannot simply relax and watch the surgery. It is a shame if you are made to feel like this, but at least you should be happier in the knowledge that you are performing useful activities. If you do these kinds of jobs, always check first that the scrub nurse has a circulator near, or one whose eye he or she can easily catch. Always be aware of what is happening at the operating table; train your senses to be constantly on the alert, even if you are involved in another activity.

It is difficult to describe the role of the circulating nurse. It involves so much. This attempt to anatomize its constituent parts still falls far short of the reality. One thing is certain – you will not realize the full importance of the circulator until you have been a scrub nurse!

Further reading

Kaczmarowski N. (1982). *Patient Care in The Operating Room.* Carlton Victoria: Pitman.

Groah, L.K. (1983). *Operating Room Nursing; The Perioperative Role.* Reston, Virginia: Prentice Hall.

9

The role of the scrub nurse

Scrubbing up to assist with surgery is what is widely considered to be the sole and proper work of the theatre nurse. The traditional image of the scrub nurse is of being at the centre of the action, controlling the team and the course of the operation, and all of this with a steely calm. Indeed it is an image to which many interested in the work aspire.

There is some truth in this image. The scrub nurse should exert some control over the theatre atmosphere, particularly over the noise level and the number of personnel present. It is also best if he or she can remain calm. These are secondary considerations however to the common aims shared with the circulating nurse. First and foremost the scrub nurse is a professional nurse concerned with the safety of patients and staff, the maintenance of asepsis and facilitating and co-ordinating the work of the surgical team.

You will no doubt be invited to scrub up at some point in your theatre experience. You can accept or refuse as you like, but it would be a pity not to take the opportunity to try out a new experience. If you are not asked soon enough for your own liking, there is no harm in taking the initiative and asking. Trained staff are always pleased to help a keen and interested student. Take their advice as to which operation you should scrub up for. They know best what is suitable, and which surgeon is more amenable to working with new students and making the experience interesting for them. It is best to scrub up for a procedure you have seen before, with a tray of instruments with which you are familiar. An ideal opportunity is a list of several of the same operations; you can watch a couple first, paying particular attention to the scrub nurse, and then have a go yourself. It is even better if you scrub up as an assistant to the surgeon first of all. This way you have an excellent view of the anatomy and the procedure and a taste of what it is like to be scrubbed up before too much is demanded of you. The first time you are a scrub nurse, you might feel more secure if one of the trained staff 'double-scrubs' with you. This removes that awful feeling of isolation, where no one can help show you how to handle things, except in dumb show, out of reach. Even if the second person simply stands there and does nothing, it is a comfort to know that real help is at hand if needed.

PREPARING IN ADVANCE

The better prepared you are, the less nervous you will be, and the operation will go more smoothly and hold more interest for you. As all operating lists should reach the department on the previous afternoon, there is no reason why you should not 'book' your case with the trained staff. This gives you the chance to read up ahead on the relevant anatomy and physiology, the operative procedure, and provides ample time to find out what your particular surgeon uses for the job. Most theatres keep records of different surgeons' requirements.

On the day of the operation, check that you have put everything you will need out ready for the circulating nurse; sutures, blades, lotions etc. Check that your tray of instruments is at hand to be opened while you scrub up; and above all, give yourself plenty of time. It is usual to begin scrubbing up when your patient has been sent for, but if you want more time, take it.

SCRUBBING UP

Before you begin, make sure that you are correctly and comfortably dressed. Is your mask securely tied? Are there any locks of hair just about to slide out from under your hat into your eyes? Have you removed your wedding ring and pinned it securely inside your pocket? It is important to see to all these things before you begin, as once you are scrubbed up you cannot put them right. You will have to rely on the help of others, which can be awkward or embarrassing. Check that a gown and gloves are open for you, and then begin.

Scrubbing up does not render you hands sterile, but should remove harmful bacteria. You will find a selection of soaps and soap solutions to choose from, which are all equally effective. Time will tell which is most suitable for your skin, so experiment with them. The taps and soap dispensers are all operated with your elbows, so start off by regulating the taps until the water is a comfortable temperature. The whole procedure should take about 4 minutes. You can time yourself initially.

Start by giving your hands a good, thorough wash, working from the tips of the fingers downwards towards the heel of the hand. Always work in this direction, letting the water run downwards from the hands to drain off at the elbows. The reason for this is that you want your fingers and hands to be the cleanest part of you, as it is these which will touch the wound. So you always work from the cleanest area to the less clean elbows, and never the other way round. Then take a scrubbing brush from the dispenser, which is again operated by the elbow, and give your fingernails a good scrub until they are clean. Then discard the brush into the appropriate container. Soap you hands again, and this time work the soap down the arms towards the elbows. Again, let the water run down over the hands and arms, draining off at the elbows. Spend the remainder of the 4 minutes really working on your hand and forearms. Always take care not to touch any other surfaces accidentally with your hands, such as the sides of the sink or the taps. If you do, you will have re-contaminated yourself, and will need to extend your scrubbing-up time to compensate.

When you have finished, switch off the water and let your arms drip-dry for a few seconds. It is safest now to keep your clean hands clasped together and your elbows well up above waist level. The area below the waist is considered unclean, a potential source of contamination. This applies throughout the period in which you are scrubbed up for the operation. Take one of the paper towels from the gown pack and dry one hand and arm, again working from the fingers downwards. Dispose of the wet towel into the pedal bin provided, operated by the feet. Repeat for the other arm.

Now you are ready to put on your *gown*. Pick the gown up off its paper, and hold it in the air well away from any furniture. Find the collar, and holding this, let the gown drop open to its full length. Gowns are always packed inside out. The part you are holding is the side which will be worn next to your theatre clothing, leaving the side which will touch the trolley drapes and the sterile field protected within. Find the outside edges of the collar and gently shake, so that now the gown is fully opened out, ready to be put on. Just before you do, have a quick look to

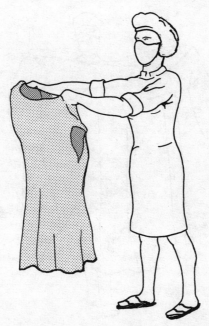

Fig. 9.1   Gowning

see that there are no holes in it. If there are, the gown will not
provide a sterile surface, and should be discarded immediately.
Slip your arms into the sleeves, but keep your hands tucked inside
the cuffs. The circulating nurse will pull the gown on more
securely for you, using the back tapes, which he or she will then
tie (Figs 9.1 and 9.2).

You are now ready to put on your *gloves*. (If you are unsure of
your glove size, try on any unsterile gloves opened in error, or
else let the trained staff make an experienced guess.) The method
of gloving described here is the 'closed method', the simplest and
safest. Open out the inner glove pack on the sterile gown paper,
still keeping your hands inside the cuffs, so that the gloves are
fully exposed. Take the left hand glove and lay it flat on your
left palm (still inside the cuff). The folded cuff of the glove should
be opposite the tips of your fingers and the fingers of the glove
facing downwards into the palm of your hand (Fig. 9.3). You
should find that your thumb and the thumb of the glove are
opposite one another, separated still by the cuff. Grasp the lip of
the folded cuff of the gloves, using your thumb and forefinger
through the gown. With the other hand (still inside its cuff) grasp

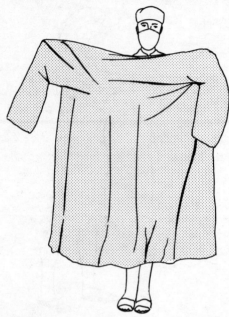

Fig. 9.2   Gowning

the lip of the glove cuff facing uppermost, and lift it right up and over the cuffed left hand. Thus the hand is sealed in, and no part of the skin touches the ouside surface of the glove; this is why this is termed the 'closed method.'

Ease the glove on, sliding the fingers into place by gently pulling the cuff of the gown downwards. (It is easier to adjust them once both hands are gloved.) Repeat the procedure for the right hand, placing the glove on the palm in the same manner and matching up the thumbs. Flip the glove over the end of the cuff using the left hand. The whole of the cuff area of the gown should be covered by glove, and it should feel comfortable, with no tight wrinkles. Remember to keep your hands well up above waist level. It is a good idea to take a pair of gloves home with you to practise if you have difficulty with the procedure.

All that remains to be done is to close the back of your gown so that your entire body is wrapped beneath a sterile surface. This has to be done with the help of someone else who has scrubbed up. On your right hand side, at about waist level, you will see two further ties on the gown, knotted together. Make sure that the ends of these ties are not dangling below knee level.

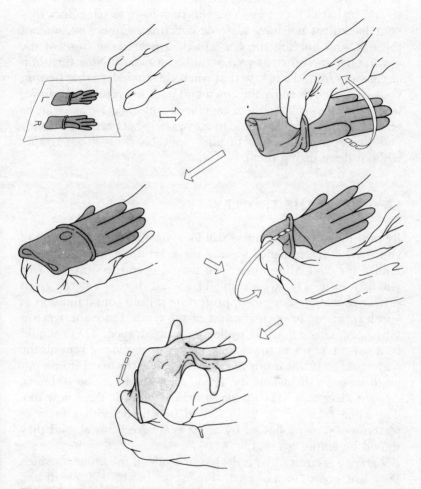

Fig. 9.3 The closed method of gloving
From *Illustrated Handbook of Minor Surgery and Operative Technique* by
Michael Saleh and Vijak Sodera (Heinemann Medical Books, 1988).
Reproduced by kind permission of the authors.

If they are, they are considered potentially contaminated, and should be left as they are. (You will then have to remember that your back does not have a sterile covering.) Otherwise, unknot the ties, and holding the one attached nearer the front of the gown, offer the other to your scrubbed assistant. Now turn in a circle away from the ties, so that when you again face that person, your back is covered by the gown and both ties meet at the front, where again you knot them together. You are now as clean as you possibly can be, and able to move safely between your trolley and the operating table, turning your back on green drapes without desterilizing them.

LAYING UP THE TROLLEY

By now the circulating nurse will have opened the inner wrap of your tray of instruments, leaving the green towel wrap exposed. Unlike the circulating nurse, you should open the wrap towards you first, instead of away from you, so that there is a sterile green surface touching your gown, protecting it from contamination as you lean across to open the rest of the wrap. Once the wrap is fully open, check that the trolley is amply draped. There should be a curtain of green towel that hangs down about 45 cm all the way around. If this is not the case, use an extra towel from your set to make up the deficiency. If you are going to use bowl stands, other trolleys or a Mayo table, it is best to drape these now too. The same rules apply. Each should be draped with a layer of waterproof paper followed by at least one green towel, and they should be amply covered.

Arrange the rest of your drapes in a pile in the order in which they are going to be used. Put your bowls, kidney dishes, instruments and swabs in order. Trained staff can usually give good advice about the layout of your trolley, helping you to make the best use of a limited working space and laying things out in the order in which they will be used. Remember though, this is your trolley; you are scrubbing up to assist with the operation. The trolley must seem comfortable and logical for you, so that you know immediately where to lay your hands on the instruments you want.

Now you are ready for your extras. Use a long pair of non-toothed forceps or a spongeholder to take the items offered by the circulating nurse, taking care not to contaminate your hands.

Take things at your own pace; do not allow the circulator to bombard you with extras too quickly. Check the skin preparation lotion with the circulating nurse and make sure that he or she also checks any other drugs to be used with the surgeon before you take them.

Having arranged everything on your trolley, you must now do your *first instrument, swab and needle count*. Remember that this must be done with a trained nurse. He or she will read out the list of instruments from the check list. You must show the nurse each item as it is called, and you must count the instruments together, out loud. Ensure everything on the check list is present; if not, double-check, and then see that the circulating nurse amends the list appropriately if the article is still not found. Any additional instruments must also be counted and added to the count sheet. Make sure that you are shown each written addition before proceeding.

Then count your swabs. Count them in bundles of five, laying each five in a separate pile. Be sure to show the Raytec markers and the tapes to your circulator, as you again count together, out loud. Open large swabs out fully to be sure that you are only counting one swab at a time. If you come across a bundle with four or six swabs in it, discard it immediately – you cannot afford to have an odd number in your count. You may like to keep the ties from the swab bundles as an extra safety check. Again check that the circulating nurse has recorded each bundle accurately on the count sheet.

Needles are counted by counting the needle symbols on each suture packet. This way you should not count any packets of ties by mistake. Take extra care if you are going to use any double-ended sutures. Any other needles, such as hypodermics, should also be counted and entered in a separate space on the count sheet. Tapes, slings and gauze rolls are counted too; slings should be separated and laid out singly as they are counted. Finally, check the count sheet again and make sure the circulating nurse has correctly entered the patient's details, both your name and his or hers, and that he or she has signed for the first count.

It is the *legal responsibility* of the scrub nurse to oversee the count to make sure that it is both performed and recorded accurately. Should anything go wrong during the operation, or if in the future the patient develops a complication as a result of negligence during the operation, such as through a swab left in the wound, the scrub nurse will be the one to go to court if litigation ensues.

When the hospital solicitor goes through the patient's notes, the count sheet will be one document retrieved in order to trace the nurses responsible for the care of that patient. In hospitals which do not use the nursing process, the count sheet may in fact be the only written record of the care delivered by the nurses in theatre. As a student nurse you will not of course be held legally responsible as the scrub nurse; that responsibility rests with the trained nurse performing the count with you. But you will soon be a trained nurse, and should appreciate that you will then be fully accountable for the care you give. So in your own interests, as well as safeguarding the health of your patient, learn to be pedantic about performing counts and checking documentation.

Another legal responsibility of the scrub nurse is to check that the right patient is about to be operated on, and that the patient has consented to the operation about to be performed. The nurse or ODA in the anaesthetic room should bring the consent form through for you to see before the operation and you should also have the circulating nurse show you the patient's wristband before the drapes go on.

INTRODUCING YOURSELF

If you have not scrubbed up before, or not scrubbed up for this particular operation or surgeon, you will feel a lot better if you say so. Ask the trained staff to introduce you to the surgeon, or take the initiative and introduce yourself. Tell the surgeon how long you have been in the department, and at what stage you are in your general training. This will be appreciated. The surgeon will know your name when he or she wants to ask you for something; you will have given some idea of the kind of help that can be expected from you; and the surgeon will have an idea of how much teaching will have to be done in order to make the operation interesting and meaningful for you. You will now feel more comfortable about the forthcoming operation, knowing that the ice has been broken.

Once the anaesthetist is happy that the patient is comfortably settled and the circulating nurse has done the safety checks, you too must observe the patient. This is because the legal responsibility for the patient's safety always devolves upon the scrub nurse, as the nursing staff representative. Check the patient's position, seeing that there is no danger of developing pressure sores or any damage to nerve pathways. Also see that the diathermy plate is correctly positioned and that the patient is not in contact with any other metal surfaces which could give rise to diathermy burns. Once you are satisfied, you can move your trolleys and other equipment into the theatre. Usually, except in orthopaedics, you need to stand on the opposite side of the table to the surgeon. Establish where he or she wants to be, and then move into position. It is also usual for, you to stand facing the patient's feet, unless this is a perineal or lower bowel operation, such as an abdominoperineal excision of rectum.

SKIN PREPARATION

The first thing you will do is to hand the surgeon the receiver of skin cleaning lotion and the mounted spongeholders. He or she will clean the skin thoroughly, working from the area where the incision is to be made outwards, covering a large surrounding area of skin. For example, if it is an abdominal operation, the surgeon will clean from the level of the patient's nipples to the groin. If it is a knee operation, the area cleansed will extend from mid-thigh down to the toes. The reason for preparing such large areas of skin is so that any adjustment necessary to the incision, and consequently the drapes, can be made safely on adequately prepared skin. If the surgeon had not prepared enough skin, the operation would have to be started all over again.

DRAPING

In draping the patient's body for surgery, the surgeon has several considerations in mind. Primarily, the aim is to create a large sterile field around the operation site on which to work. This reduces the danger of introducing infection to the wound from the atmosphere, and also protects the wound from contamination arising from other areas of the patient's own body. Only the area of skin to be operated on is to be uncovered, and the drapes should be secure enough to preserve the sterile field. This is particularly important when draping limbs, as a certain amount of manipulation is often necessary during the operation.

The following are a few of the most common ways of draping.

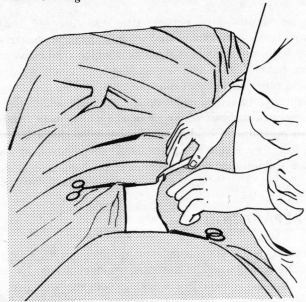

Fig. 9.4 'Square' drape

The 'square' or abdominal drape

A sheet of waterproof paper is positioned below the level of incision and over the pubic region – a possible potent source of contamination. A large drape is placed over this, covering all of the lower part of the patient's body, including the feet. A large drape is positioned above the level of incision, covering the top part of the body and the head. Two small side towels are then put into position close to the lateral margins of the incision, and secured with four towel clips (Fig. 9.4).

This type of 'square' drape can be modified for use in a variety of operations: those on the breast, the male genitalia and for kidney and back operations. In the last two cases, the patient will be lying laterally and prone respectively, so extra care needs to be taken to secure the drapes.

The neck drape

The patient will be in the supine position, with the head resting on a head ring. A sandbag may also be positioned under the shoulders for further extension of the neck.

A head towel needs to be made up to isolate the wound from

the nose, mouth and hair – potential sources of contamination. A head towel consists of a sheet of waterproof paper covered by two small drapes, opened out in full. Before the skin is prepared, the head towel is slipped into position under the patient's head, with the waterproof paper next to the operating table. (The anaesthetist will lift the head.) After cleaning, the uppermost small towel is wrapped over the patient's face and endotracheal tube from just below the level of the chin. This is secured by a towel clip. Another sheet of waterproof paper is placed on the chest, followed by a large drape to cover the whole of the lower part of the patient's body. Two small side drapes are positioned on either side of the neck, and these are secured by four towel clips.

The arm drape

The patient will be lying supine, with the affected arm lying on an arm board or table. The circulating nurse will hold the arm up in the air, by the hand, while the skin is cleaned. After cleaning, a sheet of waterproof paper is placed over the armboard, followed by a large drape; this creates a large sterile field on which to work. A small 'shut off' drape is then wrapped around the arm above the level of incision, and clipped. Another small drape is similarly applied to the hand. The surgeon will hold this drape open as the circulating nurse gently lowers the limb, and then drops the hand on to the towel, so that it is not contaminated by him or her. This towel is also clipped in place. A large drape covers the rest of the patient's body from head to toe. An additional small drape may be needed for the feet.

The knee drape

Like the arm, the leg has to be suspended by the toes during cleaning. A sheet of waterproof paper is placed under the leg, followed by a large drape to cover the other leg and the bottom end of the operating table. A small 'shut off' drape is passed under the leg, and wrapped around the area above the knee. This is clipped. The leg can then be lowered on to another small drape, which wraps around the foot and below-knee area, and this is also clipped. Alternatively, a stockinette roll can also be placed over the foot and rolled up the leg to cover the drape below the knee, and clipped. This makes the draping more secure

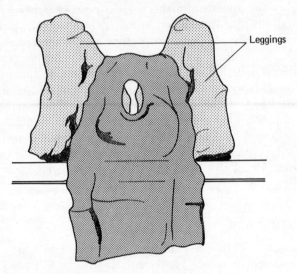

Leggings

Fig. 9.5   Perineal drape

and able to withstand manipulation of the knee joint. A large drape is put over the upper part of the patient's body.

The perineal drape

The patient will be in the lithotomy position. A sheet of waterproof paper is slid under the patient's bottom before the perineum is cleaned. Once this is done, the two leggings are put on, followed by the perineal towel with the hole in it, to isolate whichever part of the perineum is to be operated on. Finally, a large drape is used to cover the top part of the patient's body (Fig. 9.5).

These are guidelines to the methods of draping you will most commonly meet. Remember what you are trying to achieve; a large sterile field on which to work, making sure that all of the patient, other than the operation site, is covered up; good access to the site of operation, and secure drapes to preserve the sterile field.

HANDLING DRAPES

Handling drapes may pose a few problems when you are unused to them. Paper sheets should be opened out to their full width;

you should hand one end to the surgeon. Together you will open the paper out lengthways, and place it gently on top of the patient, taking care to touch nothing but the paper. It is acceptable to hand small drapes still folded up. With large drapes, as with the paper sheets, you need to find the two ends which will open the drape out to its full width. Again pass one end to the surgeon and one to the surgeon's assistant, if there is one; if not, keep hold of it yourself. You then need to locate the two edges of the drape which will open it out lengthways, and do this simultaneously with the surgeon. When the surgeon is happy with the position, let the top end of the drape drop gently into position, followed by the bottom end.

Drapes are very large unwieldy things, and because of this you must take extra care not to desterilize them. Be careful of equipment and personnel standing near the table, and be careful not to desterilize yourself. Remember that the table and patient are not sterile, so stand well back as you drape. Extra care needs to be taken when draping limbs, where drapes have to be passed under them. Take care not to desterilize yourself or the drape on the person holding the limb or on the patient's skin.

STERIDRAPES

For some operations the surgeon may wish to use a steridrape. This is a clear, adhesive drape which covers the area over the incision before surgery begins. If one is used where there is no gravitational pull on the drapes, such as for an abdominal operation, no towel clips are required; the steridrape will hold everything in place. Instead, hand the surgeon a large swab with which to dry the skin, so that the steridrape will stick. Remove the drape's loose paper covering, and find the two non-adhesive edges. Give one each to the surgeon and assistant. You then peel back the waxed lining paper, revealing the adhesive surface, which the surgeon then smooths into place.

The advantages of steridrapes are that they avoid possible damage to the skin from towel clips, but more importantly, they protect the wound edges from drying and retractor abrasions, and reduce the likelihood of infection. (At the end of operation, they must be removed from the drapes and disposed of before the linen drapes are sent to the laundry. Once exposed to the high temperatures in the washing machines, they melt and are impossible to remove. The scrub nurse should do this with gloves on, as the steridrapes are normally soiled with blood.)

The surgeon is now ready to begin, but there are still a couple of things which you need to do first. Make sure that your trolleys are comfortably in place, and that everything you need is within easy reach. You must then set up the diathermy. No skin incisions should be made until you have the means of controlling any bleeding at hand. Clip the quiver to the drapes, where both you and the surgeon have easy access to it, and pass the end of the diathermy lead out to the circulating nurse. Place the diathermy forceps inside the quiver and secure the length of sterile lead to the drapes with a towel clip. Suction tubing and any other leads you might need should also be connected now, and securely anchored to the drapes. (The quiver is also a useful place for keeping the sucker head.) Place two appropriate sized swabs ready on either side of the incision site, and then you can pass the scalpel so that surgery can begin. It is a good idea to try and keep only two swabs on the table at any one time, for ease of location.

To make a description of the role of the scrub nurse easier, let us imagine that this is an abdominal operation, and discuss the actions which constitute the scrub nurse's contribution to this specific type of surgery.

Once the skin has been incised, you should remove the skin knife and hand the surgeon the inside knife for the subcuticular and subsequent tissue layers. There are two reasons for this. Firstly, the skin is tough, and will have blunted the knife edge. Secondly, a clean knife prevents any bacteria still present on the skin from being transferred into the wound. Have the diathermy forceps ready in your hand, as the surgeon will need to coagulate bleeding points. A pair of toothed dissecting forceps will also be required to aid dissection. The surgeon will next need two strong artery forceps, usually Spencer Wells, to grip the abdominal muscle sheath as it is incised. Sometimes the surgeon will use the heavy curved Mayo scissors for this, rather than a knife, and less commonly, cutting diathermy may be used.

Once the peritoneum has been reached, you should discard all heavy and toothed instruments, replacing them with longer, finer, non-toothed ones. Remember to change the diathermy forceps too. From now on, only small swabs mounted on spongeholding forceps should be used along with large taped swabs. Now that the wound is deep, the danger of losing unmounted small swabs is too great. Large retractors will be required now to maintain good access to the operation site.

Once this access has been secured, your role as scrub nurse will be responding to the particular needs of this operation. Uppermost in your list of priorities is to provide speedy help in the control of bleeding. Make sure that there are always two clean swabs available, discarding the soaked ones into the swab bowl as you go along, and that the diathermy forceps are always at hand. It is also useful to have appropriate-length artery forceps in your hand at all times, and one in a position that is easily accessible to the surgeon. Suction too is vital for controlling more copious bleeding, so see that this is also available, and unblocked.

Try to keep the instruments tidy, so that you can find and count them easily; and clean, so that they are not bloody and slippery. Once finished with, instruments should not be left lying on the drapes, as this is how they get lost and dropped on the floor. Ask the surgeon and assistant always to pass things back to you. Be especially careful not to leave heavy instruments lying unnecessarily on the patient, or sharps, such as needles or blades. These could not only injure the patient through the drapes, but also desterilize the operative field. Never lean on the patient yourself, or allow others to! This may sound ludicrous, but it is amazing the number of people who, once they get engrossed in the operation, tend to forget there is a real, live patient under the drapes.

Remember to count groups of five discarded swabs with the circulating nurse, and to tell him or her if any swabs are tucked inside the wound. The circulator can then record this information on the swab board to remind you to retrieve the swab when closure of the wound begins. Advise him or her not to weigh swabs soaked in any substance other than blood, as this will render the estimated total of blood loss inaccurate.

Watch the depth at which the surgeon is working, and try to hand instruments of an appropriate length for the job. Remember that ties will need to be mounted on artery forceps for deep work. When needles are used, always be sure that they are returned to you, or that you know of their whereabouts if they are still attached to the wound, before you give out another needle. Remember to hand-over suture-cutting scissors to the assistant when any suturing is done. Above all, watch closely what the surgeon is doing. This is how you will learn to anticipate what is needed, not by busying yourself too much with the instruments.

Once the operative procedure is complete, and the surgeon is preparing to close the wound, you must tidy your trolley in readiness for the *first closing count*. As you did before the operation, you must count all the instruments, swabs and needles, together out loud with your circulating nurse. When you are satisfied that everything is present, you must tell the surgeon that the count is correct. He or she must acknowledge this, as the safety of the patient is ultimately the surgeon's responsibility. If it is not correct, repeat the count. If it is still not correct, you must inform the surgeon immediately, so that he or she can stop closing the wound, and a thorough search for the missing item can be instigated (see Chapter 8). All theatre nurses find it difficult to be insistent about this at first, but you must not allow yourself to be intimidated. It is vitally important that the surgeon knows something is missing and that the correct steps are taken to ensure the safety of the patient. In being insistent, you are discharging your role responsibly, laying the onus on the surgeon to take action. If you are ever the scrub nurse for an operation where the count is not complete, and the missing item is never retrieved, you must fill in an incident form. Make a photocopy of this and of the count sheet to keep for your own protection, just in case there are future repercussions.

As was noted in the previous chapter, two counts are normally done; one when the first cavity is being closed, and one when skin is sutured. This is just a guide however, meant for major surgery. Do as many or as few as you like, so long as you and the circulating nurse are both absolutely sure that everything has been accounted for and the patient is not at risk. When you are satisfied, you can tell the circulating nurse that all the used swabs can be taken down from the rack.

While performing your counts, you must also be aware of the surgeon's progress, handing over the correct sutures in the correct order for closure, and remembering to give heavier, shorter instruments to use as the operation progresses to the outer layers of tissue. Check that the surgeon has adequate swabs. Before embarking on the counts, it is a good idea to lay your closure sutures out in the order in which they are to be used. Open the foil packets ready for use, and mount some of the sutures on needleholders.

As the surgeon approaches the skin layer, ask what dressing is required. Once the final count is done, you can have this ready on the trolley along with any necessary drainage devices. Have a clean swab soaked in water or saline ready to clean the wound, and a clean dry one for drying. Once the wound is closed, you can disconnect the diathermy and suction equipment, but do ask the surgeon before you do this. When you have retrieved the last few instruments and the skin suture, hand over the cleaning swabs and then the dressing and drainage bottles.

After the operation, the scrub nurse is the best person to *accompany the patient to recovery*. As the circulating nurse cares for the patient immediately after the drapes are removed, you can cover and push your trolley out to the sluice area. You can check it again once the patient is safely despatched. As the scrub nurse, you have a better knowledge of the operative procedure, and know precisely what dressings and drains have been used. You are therefore able to give a better, more detailed handover to the recovery nurses than your circulator could, and to ensure that your patient receives a consistently high standard of care.

Before leaving the theatre, first of all check the comfort and safety of the patient, and see that the anaesthetist has all that is necessary. Be sure that you have all the relevant paperwork; the patient's notes, x-rays, anaesthetic sheet, drug chart and the completed count sheet. Now you can give all your attention to assisting the anaesthetist to care for the patient's airway. *The maintenance of a clear and effective airway is everyone's top priority* until the patient has recovered sufficiently from the anaesthetic to do this independently. Where there is particular concern about a patient's airway, portable suction can be attached to the bed for use on the journey between the theatre and recovery room. This is especially useful if the two areas are far apart. Always be aware of other suction apparatus in the departments you pass which could be used in an emergency, such as that kept in a vacant anaesthetic room. It is also vital to know how to tip the patient's trolley in case vomiting occurs. (When the patient is transferred to the trolley from the operating table, be sure that he or she is lying the correct way round, so that this will be possible.)

In recovery you can facilitate the delivery of the recovery nurse's care by helping to arrange the patient comfortably, together with any other necessary equipment. Remember that the recovery nurse will have to hold the patient's jaw initially to maintain a clear airway, so another pair of hands is most welcome. You are the one who can find her a dripstand, and who can hang up the catheter bag and any other drainage bags where they are clearly visible. The anaesthetist will hand over information about the anaesthetic, the patient's vital signs, oxygen and drug therapy and any postoperative intravenous fluid regimes. You explain about the operation, and together with the recovery nurse, you should inspect the dressing and drainage bottles for any oozing, to establish a baseline observation from which to work. Point out any other appendages, such as nasogastric tubes or catheters, and be sure to pass on any special instructions from the surgeon. Before leaving recovery, do just double-check that all the paperwork is present and correct. It is time-consuming and frustrating for the recovery nurse to have to chase up missing documents.

Then you can sort out your trolley. All disposable materials should be removed from the set and placed in the rubbish bag. Sharps are dealt with separately. Make sure that nothing sharp, such as blades, needles or ampoules, remains on the set. Failure to do this could result in the injury of one of the TSSU staff, and place them at risk of contracting a blood-borne infection. These items must all be discarded into the sharps bin, or else placed inside a special, sealing disposal pad, which is safe to put in with the ordinary rubbish. Linen is discarded into the linen skip, and you can then tie up all the disposal bags, ready for removal from the department. Sorting out the rubbish may not seem a very glamorous task but it is an important one, and one which must be done responsibly. You must consider the health and safety of colleagues as well as your own. Gloves must be worn throughout the procedure.

Finally, check your set of instruments once more, and indicate on the check list that they are all present. See that all the other relevant details have also been entered correctly – the patient's name, your name and the theatre number – before closing up the drapes, leaving the list tucked just inside, where the TSSU staff will be able to find it. Any additional instruments must be dealt with according to department policy, either returning them separately to TSSU or else washing and preparing them to be packed by nursing staff.

The final responsibility of the scrub nurse is to ensure that the *theatre documentation* has been properly completed. Every theatre has a register of operations, usually kept in the anaesthetic room. Again, this is a very important legal document, recording exactly what happened and who was present. Along with the count sheet, this is the other piece of evidence signed by nursing staff declaring that all was well. See that the patient's details were correctly entered by the ward nurse, and then fill in the name of the operative procedure. No abbreviations are acceptable; everything must be written out in full so that there is no room for ambiguity or speculation. The names of the surgeon, assistant and anaesthetist must be entered, along with details of the type of anaesthetic given – local or general. Finally, you must sign your name, indicating that you were the scrub nurse, and see that your circulating nurse countersigns. These are the basic facts which must be established in the register. It cannot be over-emphasized that everything must be accurately stated and signed for.

Most students enjoy scrubbing up for operations. Their theatre experience suddenly becomes more interesting and they feel more personally involved in the care of the patient. If you gain nothing else from the experience, you will at least appreciate the need for the services of a good, reliable circulating nurse, and gain insight into how to improve your own performance in this role. Never forget to thank your back-up team!

Further reading

MDU and RCN (1978). *Safeguards Against Wrong Operations* and *Safeguards against Failure to Remove Swabs and Instruments from Patients*. Joint Memoranda, London: MDU and RCN.
Dixon E. (1984). *The Theatre Nurse and the Law*, Kent: Croom Helm.

10

Recovery

As in anaesthetics, this is another area where you will probably
feel more at home. The equipment is more familiar, and you
have the satisfaction of caring for your patient on a one-to-one
basis. Almost all patients spend some time in recovery, regardless
of whether they have had a general or local anaesthetic. This
allows time for them to wake up, to be fully in control of their
airway and to show a stable, satisfactory set of vital signs. They
return to the wards fully oriented in time and space, when the
danger of any immediate postoperative complication has passed.
The ward nurses therefore receive back patients who have made
an initial recovery from surgery in a stable and satisfactory
condition.

As elsewhere in the department, it is essential that you are
fully oriented to the area before undertaking to care for any
postoperative patients. The recovery room consists of several bays
or spaces for the patient's trolleys, each equipped for recovery
(see Chapter 2, for a description of the equipment). Make sure
that you know how to operate the oxygen supply, and where to
find fresh masks and tubing. These are changed for each patient.
If cylinders of oxygen are used, make sure that you know where
spares can be obtained. You should also know where the small,
portable cylinders are located – the ones which are mounted on
to patients' beds, should they need to continue therapy after
leaving recovery. Make sure you know how to operate the suction,
and where to obtain fresh tubing, suction heads and catheters.
Again, these are changed for every patient.

You need to locate the emergency trolley, with the defibrillator
and tray of intubation equipment (see Chapter 5 for a description
of intubation equipment). You need to know how to tip the
trolleys to clear the airway of a vomiting patient. It is vital that
you know these things; but there is a host of other things of lesser
importance which you should also know. Just to mention a few,
you need to locate: vomit bowls, tissues, bedpans, bottles, screens,
extra linen, dressings, the drug cupboard, the telephone and the

recovery register. You will be oriented to the area by the trained staff, and you can also make use of the extra time available in the mornings when surgery is getting underway, for this purpose.

Before recovering a patient on your own, you will initially be working with or observing one of the trained nurses in action. *When patients have had a general anaesthetic, caring for and maintaining the airway is the top priority.* When they arrive in recovery, they will be given oxygen via a face mask or nasal cannulae. Once this is in place, the recovery nurse takes over from the anaesthetist in supporting the angles of the patient's jaw. This extends the neck and prevents the tongue obstructing the airway. Thus the patient receives the full benefit of the oxygen. You must practise holding the jaw under supervision, as it is vital to the patient's safety. Oxygen therapy and a clear airway are always established before taking any handovers from the anaesthetist or scrub nurse.

The anaesthetist's handover will consist of a description of the anaesthetic and information about the patient's observations throughout surgery, which will give you a baseline for comparison. Make sure that all of this has been adequately recorded. If an intravenous infusion is in situ, make sure that it is dripping, and that a postoperative intravenous fluid regime has been prescribed. (When your hands are free from holding the patient's jaw, you should also inspect the infusion site.) The oxygen should also have been prescribed, along with postoperative analgesics and anti-emetics. You should establish whether or not the anaesthetist wishes to see the patient again before he or she is returned to the ward.

From the scrub nurse, you need to find out details of the operative procedure, again checking that this information has been adequately recorded. Together you should inspect the dressings for any signs of oozing or primary haemorrhage, and also any drainage bottles, catheter bags or bile bags attached. Only when you are entirely happy that you understand what has happened, that the patient's condition presents no immediate problems and that you have adequate prescriptions and any special instructions, should you allow the anaesthetist and scrub nurse to leave.

Begin to reassure and orient your patient straight away; both of these things are needed, together with the stimulation of your voice and touch. It is only usually a matter of up to 10 minutes before patients are awake enough to spit out the Magill airway. You can encourage them to do this, but never pull the airway out yourself. Until the patient is able to expel it independently, he or she is probably not capable of maintaining the airway adequately. There is also the danger that in pulling on the airway you could damage crowns or caps on teeth. This could not only be annoying and possibly expensive for the patient, but could have dangerous consequences if dislodged and inhaled. When the Magill airway is out, you no longer need to hold the patient's jaw. Before replacing the face mask, you should explain to the patient that this is a means of delivering oxygen, and it must stay in place until the patient is more fully awake. Your hands are now free to carry out other observations, unless you have an assistant who has been doing them for you. Remember that care of the airway always comes first; other observations can wait.

How can you tell if the airway is not clear? What signs are you looking for? The cardinal sign of a blocked airway is the absence of chest movement. You must observe the patient constantly for chest expansion and relaxation, and the misting of the exhaled breath on the oxygen mask. When holding the jaw you can also feel the exhaled breath on the heel of your hand. Watch out for any changes in the respiratory rate too. Before the patient stops breathing altogether, the breaths may become laboured, more irregular and inadequate.

The second most important thing to observe is the patient's colour – a very sensitive indicator of the state of the airway. If this is blocked, the patient's skin colour will deepen to dark red, purple and then blue, at a fairly rapid rate. A completely blocked airway is silent, but any unusual breathing sounds also indicate a degree of obstruction. If the sound is rattling or bubbly, there are loose secretions in the airway; but if the noise is a tight, high-pitched gasping, this indicates laryngospasm.

Whatever the signs are which tell you that the airway is blocked, you must act quickly to reverse the situation. Summon trained help immediately. If the patient is not already on the side in the recovery position, he or she must be turned. Then with the suction apparatus, as much mucus as possible must be removed from the mouth and pharynx. If the patient has vomited, then the trolley should be tipped head-down so that the vomit is not inhaled. (This of course is provided that the surgery just completed does not contraindicate this – such as surgery to the head, and particularly the eyes, where an increase in intracranial pressure is undesirable.) Once the aspirate has been cleared, put the Magill airway back into position and continue to give oxygen. These measures are usually adequate to clear the airway, restoring a healthy colour and respirations. If not, the trained staff will call the anaesthetist back. There may be several factors influencing the patient's inability to maintain spontaneous respiration, which can only be resolved by re-intubation or drug therapy or a combination of both. The patient's respiratory centre may be depressed due to an excess of narcotics still in circulation. Inability to breathe properly may be due to inadequate reversal of muscle relaxants, which continue to inhibit respiratory muscular activity. The patient may also be experiencing an allergic reaction to one of the anaesthetic agents or postoperative drugs.

Once the patient is breathing spontaneously without an airway, you can carry out observations of blood pressure and pulse which, along with those of respirations, are recorded on the anaesthetic chart. Initially these are done at least every quarter of an hour, but less frequently as recordings stabilize in a satisfactory manner. If you are unhappy with an observation, check back through the anaesthetist's recordings, both during surgery and preoperatively. It may be normal for the patient to have high blood pressure. If there is little correlation between these readings and your own, check the reading again after a couple of minutes. If you are still unhappy, summon trained help.

As part of your observations, do not forget to check the running of intravenous infusions or other types of irrigation, or to check the patient's dressings and drains. Report anything you are worried about, particularly if there is any bleeding at the site of operation. Dressings may need to be changed, or extra padding added to exert pressure on the wound.

Continually reassure the patients, and explain every procedure before you carry it out. Now that they are more awake, you can ask them how they feel. They will no doubt be feeling some pain and possibly nausea, which you can relieve. Provided that the blood pressure is not too low, they can be given intramuscular injections of an analgesic and anti-emetic. Emphasize that the operation is over (many won't believe you) and remind them that they are in recovery, and that shortly a nurse will be coming to take them back to the ward. At some stage, when you feel it is safe enough to walk away from the patient for a few moments, you will need to enter the details in the recovery register.

When the patient is awake, oriented, comfortable, and the observations are stable, it is time for the patient to go back to the ward. Until you are more experienced and confident about your decisions here, it is a good idea to get one of the trained staff to assess the patient as well. You may also now need to call the anaesthetist back, before telephoning the ward, if he or she expressed a wish to see the patient again.

Before the ward nurse arrives, check that you have gathered together the patient's notes, x-rays, anaesthetic chart, drug chart and any other necessary paperwork. See that you have completed the recovery notes fully. Check that the patient is ready to be moved, and not going back to the ward with any theatre or recovery equipment still attached. Heel supports and blood pressure cuffs frequently go missing in this way. Have you removed all unnecessary intravenous cannulae, such as butterflies in the back of the hand? (Never do this without having asked the anaesthetist first. Most butterflies can be removed, but occasionally the anaesthetist may wish to leave one access open.)

When the ward nurse arrives, the patient will be moved to the transfer bay, and lifted from the theatre trolley back into bed. Help the ward nurse to make the patient safe and comfortable, and to arrange any bed equipment, such as portable oxygen cylinders. Make your handover thorough, repeating everything told to you, and adding significant information of your own. Explain the operative procedure, and indicate the written accounts of both the surgeon and scrub nurse. Showing sensitivity to the patient's dignity and understanding, you should together inspect drains, dressings and any other appendages. Explain about the anaesthetic, and show both yours and the anaesthetist's recordings of the patient's observations. Point out any problems that arose, and explain how they were dealt with. Tell the ward nurse about any intravenous infusions and oxygen therapy to be continued, indicating the appropriate prescriptions. Also indicate the analgesics and anti-emetics prescribed, and if any have been given, say at what time. Any special nursing care instructions must also be passed on. A good verbal handover, backed up with good, complete documentation, ensures continuity of a high standard of care for your patient.

This is an outline of the events which constitute a patient's initial recovery from surgery following a general anaesthetic. (The care of patients following local anaesthesia is outlined in Chapter 5.) It is only a general outline; of course details vary, depending on the nature of the operation and the anaesthetic, but the above description gives some idea of the routine care delivered by recovery nurses. A high standard of care at this vulnerable time, responding immediately to any need for further surgical or anaesthetic intervention, coupled with good communication of that care, can profoundly influence for the better the patient's subsequent recovery and prognosis.

Further reading

Stephens D.S.B., Boaler J. (1977). The nurse's role in immediate post-operative care. *Nursing Mirror,* **145** (13), pp. 20–3.
Norris W. and Campbell D. (1985). *Nurse's Guide to Anaesthetics, Resuscitation and Intensive Care* 6th ed. Edinburgh: Churchill Livingstone.

11

Pre- and postoperative visiting

Many theatre nurses today are visiting patients on the wards, both before and after surgery. This is proving invaluable for all concerned – patients, the theatre nurses themselves and ward nurses. If you have the opportunity, go and assess the value of these visits yourself. You will probably be struck by some of the following advantages.

Patients are shown a friendly human face belonging to one of those masked, faceless theatre staff. This is very reassuring, and can be especially so if the same nurse greets the patient on arrival in the operating department.

Although medical staff explain forthcoming surgery to patients, this does not always mean that patients are left feeling entirely clear about what is going to happen to them. The reason for this is usually due to the pressure of limited time. Medical staff cannot afford to spend much time with them, and the short space of time between admission and operation means that many questions remain unanswered. Patients forget information too; memory is not at its best under the stress of an impending operation (Summers, 1984).

Theatre nurses, in tandem with the ward nurses, can help considerably here. They can alleviate uncertainty and anxiety by spending time with patients reinforcing pre- and postoperative advice, and giving a fuller account of the operative procedure. A good way of discovering where help is most needed is to encourage the patient to explain his or her understanding of what is going to happen and of the consent form. In this way any misconceptions can be dealt with and extra emphasis can be given to the most important things for the patient to remember. Leaving written information for reference can help to overcome the memory difficulties.

As well as exploring a patient's understanding of the surgery about to be undergone, theatre nurses can also use their visits to ask how the patient feels about it. This is an area of concern most frequently avoided when time is short. The theatre nurse must then of course be prepared for the consequences of delving more deeply. A sympathetic listener with time on her hands may find herself the recipient of expressed fears hitherto unexplored with another human being. The fears of death under anaesthetic, of disfigurement and of the discovery of an unknown cancer are commonly felt but often left unexpressed. Theatre nurses must reassure patients as best they can and obviously, interviews that have unearthed these kinds of fears cannot be terminated abruptly and thoughtlessly. Knowing your own limitations is therefore important. Any questions relating to prognosis and future treatment should be referred to medical staff, as speculation without precise knowledge can be dangerous. Experience has shown that patients are normally considerably reassured and less anxious after being visited preoperatively by a theatre nurse (Hughes, 1979).

As well as giving psychological support, preoperative visits also enhance the physical care of patients. The theatre nurse has access to the patient's notes and nursing care plan, and thus can read about any potential physical problems. He or she can then assess the patient independently. Of particular interest will be: the condition of the patient's skin, any prostheses, deafness, obesity, chest complaints, smoking habits, previous anaesthetic problems, spastic limbs, allergies, any infections and blindness. Religious beliefs are also noted, as some will affect a patient's attitude towards surgery. Jewish patients request that any amputated limbs receive full burial rites, and Jehovah's Witnesses will not accept transfusions of blood or any blood products. Armed with all this information, the theatre nurse can plan individualized patient care in the operating department; care which will give psychological support and enhance physical and spiritual well-being.

Visiting the wards on a regular basis allows the growth of friendly personal relationships between theatre and ward nurses. This is a great improvement on the past, when contact only seemed to be made to complain about each other's mistakes or omissions. Now theatre and ward nurses have a greater appreciation of one another's roles in the care of patients, and an understanding of each other's particular problems and preoccupations. The contact made through ward visits allows for exchange of ideas and keeping abreast of policy changes too; in fact, an overall integration of high standards of care. The benefits for patients are considerable (Thompson, 1981).

Planning individualized care does mean more paper work for theatre nurses, but it has proved to be well worth it. Better, more detailed documentation of patient care in the operating department helps to ensure the continuity of that care, and provides the ward nurses with invaluable references upon which to base their own observations. The theatre nurse's entry in the patient's care plan should include the following information:

1 Type of anaesthetic.
2 Position on the table.
3 Site of diathermy pad.
4 Skin preparation lotion used.
5 Type of incision.
6 Operative procedure.
7 Verification of swab, instrument and needle counts.
8 Details of any implants, e.g. drains, catheters, infusions etc.
9 Type of dressing.
10 Any special nursing instructions from the surgeon.

The recovery nurses, experts in immediate postoperative care, can add to this their comments and any nursing care instructions which they feel will benefit the patient on the ward. A full account of care given in the operating department also benefits theatre nurses. In these days of increased litigation, it helps to constitute a good legal defence.

Legal accountability aside, pre- and postoperative visiting has had other beneficial spin-offs for theatre nurses. In the past they have worked too much in isolation from the rest of hospital life, and seen patients only in the context of their own department. Ward visits have changed all this, and given theatre nurses the chance to follow the progress of patients right through their hospital stay and to share in their broader hopes and aims in life, not just in their operation. It is very satisfying to be recognized by patients as important contributors to their care, whereas in the past there was no opportunity for this recognition to be communicated.

Postoperative visits allow theatre nurses the chance to evaluate the care they gave both pre- and peroperatively. Evaluation is based on the theatre nurse's own observations of the patient's recovery and progress, and significant contributions from patients themselves, who can pinpoint areas where physical care could be improved and highlight aspects of procedures which could be more fully explained. Postoperative visits therefore give the opportunity constantly to adapt and improve theatre nursing skills, working towards the good postoperative recovery of every patient. For the theatre manager they also provide a wealth of information, which when collated over a period of time provides the means of quality control.

For the whole system to work there has to be a lot of behind-the-scenes organization, which in itself brings benefits. Many searching questions have to be answered for a start. Why is pre- and postoperative visiting useful? What can be gained from it? Reference must be made to research publications and nursing press articles to answer this. Specific aims peculiar to that operating department then have to be identified. These may indeed vary from theatre to theatre, reflecting the type of surgery carried out in each. How are the visits to be conducted? In order to produce guidelines for staff there must be much consultation and discussion of all these issues amongst senior nurses, both in theatres and on the wards.

A burning question with regard to visiting patients is: 'Who is going to visit?' Patients need an accurate informed source of information, and someone whose rank lends authority and credibility. It has already been noted that in the past theatre nurses were isolated and not used to communicating with patients on the wards. Do they then need help with counselling and interpersonal skills? Fears of such inadequacy have proved common, and it is only by admitting and confronting these fears that beneficial change can occur. Is it desirable to leave some form of written information with patients? If so, what form should it take and how detailed should it be? When are visits to occur? Obviously the off-duty rota needs to be looked at in order to be able to release nurses to visit without seriously depleting the staff working in the department. When is it a good time for the patient? How is the information gained from visits to be communicated to the theatre team?

All these questions have presented theatre nurses with a stimulating challenge. Answering them has revolutionized theatre nursing practice. A more professional service to patients has evolved, along with personal development and increased job satisfaction for the nurses. When patients have shorter, smoother recovery periods from surgery money is also saved and it seems we must all learn to count the costs these days!

Accompanying theatre nurses on their pre- and postoperative visits and witnessing the delivery of their planned care inside the department will allow you to see the role of the theatre nurse in its entirety. Following the progress of several patients through surgery will also give you a greater appreciation of the logic behind all that is done for surgical patients, and the chance to share in patients' reactions to this care. Your surgical nursing skills will be enormously enhanced, leaving you better equipped to help patients not only in theatres, but also on the wards.

References

Hughes J. (1979). Overcoming fear: the pre-operative visit. *Nursing Times*, (Theatre Nursing Supplement) **75** (42), pp. 4–6.
Summers R. (1984). Should patients be told more? *Nursing Mirror*, **159** (7), pp. 16–20.
Thompson R. (1981). Implementing the nursing process in operating theatres. *NAT News*, **18** (10), pp. 18–24.

Further reading

Alcock P. (1986). Pre-operative information and visits promote the recovery of patients. *NAT News*, **23** (7), pp. 17–18.
Boore J. (1978). *Prescription for Recovery*, London: Royal College of Nursing.
Davis B. (1972). Tell them like it is. *Nursing Mirror*. **154** (12), pp. 26–8.
Geraghty J. (1985). Theatre nurses – the way foward. *World of Irish Nursing*. **14** (1), pp. 13–14.
Hayward J. (1985). *A Prescription against Pain*. London: Royal College of Nursing.
Kerrigan J. (1982). One theatre team's experience of pre and post-operative visits. *NAT News*. **19** (4), pp. 14–16.
Leonard M. (1984). No time to visit? *Senior Nurse*, **I**, pp. 22–3.
Shaw H. (1983). What aspects of the nursing process are applicable in theatre nursing and how can they be implemented? *NAT News*. **20** (5), pp. 11–13.

12

Dealing with infected patients

Occasionally patients with a known infection have to come to theatre for surgery. Special precautions are obviously necessary. There are three concerns here. Firstly, to protect that particular patient's wound from contamination elsewhere in the body. Secondly, to protect the clean operating department environment from contamination, which could lead to cross-infection of subsequent patients. Thirdly, to safeguard the health of operating department personnel. All infected patients should be treated with the same caution, but extra care should be taken when dealing with blood-borne infections such as hepatitis and the AIDS virus, and resistant *Staphylococcus aureus*, which is so prevalent in hospitals these days. Every department will have a *written policy* for dealing with infected patients to which you should refer. The following considerations will probably be included in the hospital policy.

Medical staff are asked to give as much *prior warning* as possible when booking an operation for a patient with an existing infection. This allows the theatre nurses to plan ahead, and to accommodate the operation where the risk of cross-infection will be minimal. Ideally, a theatre away from the mainstream of surgery should be used, and one that is not currently in use for a list of planned surgery. Failing that, infected patients should be added to the end of an operating list. This is because all theatres are cleaned thoroughly at the end of a list, and also to allow as many air changes as possible to occur before the theatre is again in use. Ideally, the theatre will now be empty overnight, but if this is not possible, it should stand empty for at least an hour.

So that minimal theatre equipment comes into contact with or is exposed to contaminated material, the chosen theatre is stripped of most of its *furniture*. Only the very basics are left inside: the diathermy machine, the suction and a stool for the anaesthetist. Anything not required for use should be pushed outside into the theatre corridor or the clean preparation room. Even the linen skip and rubbish bag frames can be removed, leaving only the disposal bags themselves inside the theatre. The swab rack can go too, being replaced by sheets of waterproof paper spread on the floor. The swabs can be arranged into groups of five on these sheets, as in the lost swab procedure. Only minimal *disposable packs* should be left inside the theatre, such as swabs and sutures, as any unused packs will still need to be discarded at the end of operation, as their outer wrappers are potentially contaminated.

It is essential to have a bare minimum of *staff* too. The scrub nurse needs one circulator inside the theatre – the 'dirty' circulator – and a 'clean' circulator in the clean preparation room to pass in any necessary equipment. All staff in the theatre must wear overshoes, a gown and gloves – this includes anaesthetic staff. The scrubbed team need to wear two pairs of gloves. As far as possible all of these will be made of disposable material. In the case of blood-borne infections, all staff in theatre must wear plastic goggles to protect their eyes from infection by blood splashes. When the operation is over, staff should change their theatre clothing before coming into contact with other patients.

The scrub nurse prepares the trolley of instruments in exactly the same way as usual, maintaining asepsis and performing all the safety checks. However disposable paper drapes will be used in place of linen where possible.

While the operation is underway, the 'clean' circulator can *prepare for the disposal of all contaminated material* at the end of the operation. A large bowl of strong disinfectant (such as sodium hypochlorite solution), disposable cleaning cloths, a mop and a bucket of the same solution are required. With these, the scrub nurse and 'dirty' circulator will wash all the instruments and clean all the theatre surfaces. Having been initially disinfected, the *instruments* will then need to be autoclaved immediately. They will travel to the TSSU in some kind of container sealed with autoclave tape, perhaps in a metal trunk or in a double layer of strong plastic bags. The 'clean' circulator will need to collect these items along with an outer disposal bag for both the rubbish and the linen. The *rubbish* bag should be clearly marked with tape: 'infected rubbish'. The porters will then know to remove it and have it sent down to the hospital incinerator as soon as possible. Most hospitals have a distinctive colour-coding for *linen* bags, so if you collect one of the correct colour for infected linen, no further labelling should be necessary. *Sharps* are best disposed of in a sealing disposal pad which can safely be put into the rubbish. If this is not available, the 'clean' circulator will also need to collect a sharps bin, which must be securely sealed afterwards and again, clearly marked: 'infected sharps'. All of this equipment can be put ready on a large trolley outside the theatre door leading to the sluice.

When the operation is over, and all the swabs and drapes are correctly bagged, the 'dirty' circulator will place these by the theatre door. Other staff leaving can then drop their overshoes, gowns, gloves and masks in as they step through the doorway. The cleaning solution is then passed in and the scrub nurse and 'dirty' circulator will now stay inside the theatre until all the surfaces have been washed and all the contaminated material passed out. The 'clean' circulator holds the outer disposal bags open ready to receive the instruments, linen and rubbish. The 'clean' circulator is responsible for securing them and again checking the labelling, and for dispatching the instruments to TSSU.

Any *specimens* taken are packaged for transit in the same way. The pot is placed inside two transparent transporter bags along with the appropriate request card. *Suction units* are cleared by sucking disinfectant solution through the tubing into the bottles. Most bottles can then be removed and autoclaved. *Anaesthetic equipment* is dealt with in the same manner as the other instruments. The nurse or ODA will wash all the items used in disinfectant; most of the equipment – such as circuit tubing, masks, and laryngoscope blades – can also be put through the autoclave, if this is deemed necessary. Finally, the disinfectant solution is poured down the theatre drains before the scrub nurse and 'dirty' circulator leave.

If such care is taken, the risk of cross-infection will be minimal. The theatre will be cleaned again by the porters or commercial cleaners in the evening, and the ventilation system will ensure many air changes before surgery is again performed.

As an extra staff safeguard, many hospitals list in the *theatre register* all those present during the operation along with details of the infection to which they have been exposed. This is often done in red ink, so that it is easier for occupational health staff making periodic checks to identify staff at risk. This is particularly effective in the case of patients suspected of an infection or in a high risk potential group, when the diagnosis may not be confirmed until after surgery.

Should any *accidents* happen, particularly where staff sustain cuts from a contaminated instrument, the nursing officer should be informed immediately and an accident form completed. The person involved will need to be seen by medical staff in the occupational health department and receive any necessary treatment. The importance of filling in an *accident form* cannot be over-emphasized. It may seem a nuisance and tedious at the time, but it is evidence that the accident occurred at work, and should your health suffer as a result, this evidence will be used to ensure that you receive any benefits or compensation to which you are entitled.

13

Health and safety matters

You will probably already have heard of the *Health and Safety at Work Act, 1974*. This is an Act of Parliament outlining the responsibilities of both employers and employees in relation to maintaining health and safety. It is an Act which applies not only to hospitals, but to all types of industry and office environments right across the board. Until 1987 hospitals enjoyed crown immunity in relation to health and safety inspectors' recommendations. This meant that they would listen to the advice given, but then could decide for themselves how far to implement change. Now they are obliged by law to comply completely with the recommendations of the health and safety inspector. Failure to do so can result in prosecution. This is a significant change, and one which requires greater awareness of health and safety issues.

To summarize the contents of the Act, it states that the maintenance of health and safety is a two-way process. Employers are responsible for deciding what constitutes a safe environment in their place of work, and then outlining safe working practices to achieve this. Thought has to be given to maintaining this level of safety, which means devising procedures to follow in the event of an emergency and a programme of routine safety checks to identify and eliminate hazards. Finally, it is also employers' responsibility to inform and train staff in the use of these procedures, constantly evaluating their effectiveness, and to promote a general awareness of the need to safeguard health and safety.

To facilitate the growth of awareness amongst the workforce, certain employees can be given extra tuition coupled with the responsibility of disseminating their knowledge. You will probably be introduced to your health and safety representative in the operating department. Within the larger framework of the hospital you are also no doubt aware of the existence of specialist health and safety officers, such as the control of infection officer, the radiological protection adviser, the fire prevention officer, the electrical safety officer and the security officer. These functions are the responsibilities of the employer.

Your responsibility as an employee is to take reasonable care of your own health and safety, and that of your colleagues. You must co-operate with the employers in pursuing the policies laid down, and not intentionally or recklessly misuse materials provided for this purpose. The responsibility of maintaining high standards of health and safety care is shared between those who create the risks and those who work with them.

When you first enter the operating department, you will probably be struck by the staff's consciousness of the need to maintain health and safety. This is not at all surprising as the operating department houses a large number of potential hazards. In order that you may carry out your side of the bargain – taking reasonable care of yourself and your colleagues – it is essential that you are aware of these hazards and understand safe working methods to minimize their potential effect. Some instruction on health and safety matters will no doubt be included in your orientation programme, but let us again identify the major hazards and discuss how to deal with them.

We have already mentioned some of the most important hazards, such as the potential for *cross-infection*, and will do so again, as this dictates almost every aspect of how we design and behave in the operating department. Procedures for dealing with infected patients are dealt with specifically in Chapter 12. The risk to staff of contracting blood-borne infections, such as hepatitis and AIDS, and how to minimize this risk, have been especially highlighted.

Fire hazards, in connection with the large amount of electrical equipment in the department, have also been mentioned in Chapter 2. Again, it must be stressed that regular safety checks and maintenance programmes for items such as the diathermy machine, suction apparatus, lights, anaesthetic monitoring equipment and portable heaters, are essential. It is your responsibility to report immediately any faulty equipment.

Fire hazards are also posed by the large amount of inflammable substances in the department. Oxygen is of course the major risk here, and don't forget that the department has a plentiful supply in all areas, either from piped sources or cylinders. The anaesthetic gas cyclopropane is also highly inflammable, but thankfully has largely been withdrawn from use these days. Occasionally a department may keep just one cylinder in its store, distinguishable by its small size and British Standard colouring of orange. Other commonly found inflammable substances are some of the volatile anaesthetic agents, such as ether.

The dangers of a build-up of *static electricity*, and its potential to cause explosions, has also been mentioned in Chapter 2. As you can see, it is vital for you to co-operate with the department management in wearing anti-static footwear and being aware of the fire-fighting equipment available. Make sure that you know the position of fire alarms, extinguishers, hoses and fire exits. You should also make it your responsibility to read the department policy on what to do in the event of fire.

Another hazard posed by the large amount of electrical equipment is the potential for staff injuries resulting from *flexes* on the floor and *badly positioned equipment*. Common sense should tell you that where possible, flexes should be positioned away from areas of great staff activity. If this is not possible, they should be adhered to the floor with sleek strapping, and there should certainly not be any tangled flexes. The same applies to the positioning of equipment; if possible it should be out of the general thoroughfare. Staff working unavoidably close to equipment which could potentially injure them must be warned. This applies particularly to the scrub team, who become so engrossed in the operation that they will often forget that a large, portable operating lamp is just behind them!

A greater number of *x-rays* are taken in the operating department than on the wards. Some types of surgery are particularly reliant on x-ray verification, such as orthopaedic trauma surgery, where the correct alignment of bones must be continually checked. Genitourinary surgery increasingly employs the use of x-rays, particularly for detecting and dislodging renal calculi. In general surgery too, the cholecystectomy and peroperative cholangiogram, to detect the presence of stones in the common bile duct, is a common operation.

Wherever you work in the operating department, you are bound to come into contact with x-rays, and should know how to protect yourself and your colleagues from their adverse effects. As you are no doubt already aware, over-exposure to x-rays can damage the cells of the ovaries and testes, leading to infertility or possibly the mutation of genes. As operating departments are largely staffed by young people who may be planning to have families in the future, it is vital that everyone is meticulous about following the safety procedures.

Lead coats are provided by the radiography department, who are normally responsible for their maintenance. These should be worn in the theatre by all personnel whenever an x-ray is taken. For an operation involving x-ray control throughout, scrubbed staff should be careful to put a lead coat on before they scrub up, wearing their sterile gown over the top. As you can imagine, this can be very uncomfortable. Wearing a lead coat for any length of time makes you very hot; they are also very heavy, making your legs and back ache. Unfortunately this is unavoidable. As when dealing with an infected case, as few staff as possible should be present; avoidance of radiation is the best strategy for the maintenance of health. Pregnant women, or those who think they might be, should not be in the theatre at all. Radiation can damage a developing fetus.

When the x-ray is taken, it is best to step back from the x-ray machine as far as possible, and better still if you can manage to interpose a wall or some other solid structure between you and it. This has the effect of diminishing the concentration of radiation you receive. If you should walk unawares into a theatre where x-rays are being taken, you can be protected by standing behind someone wearing a lead coat. This should only be done as a temporary, emergency measure however, as it is not wholly satisfactory as a means of protection.

Lead coats come in various designs. Some amply cover you front and back, provided that the side fastenings are done up. Some, however, to make them lighter and more comfortable, cover the front and only half of your back. Lead aprons only shield the pelvis. If you are wearing one of these latter two designs, remember that your back is not protected. So move accordingly, never turning your back towards the x-ray machine.

Although the radiographers normally maintain the lead coats, it is the responsibility of everyone who uses them to treat them with respect and not damage them. Immediately after use they should be hung on coat hangers. Leaving the coats crumped up cracks their lead coating, so that in future the protection they offer will be defective.

If you work in an area where many x-rays are taken regularly, you may also be given a blue radiation detection badge. You should wear this pinned on to the outside of your theatre clothing. It is in your own interest to remember to wear it at all times, as it contains a small photographic film which measures the amount of scattered irradiation to which you have been exposed. Your theatre sister will keep a record of the number badge allocated to you. Periodically the radiation protection officer will recall the badges and issue new ones, so that the films can be checked. Staff who have been exposed to high doses of radiation will be recommended for a blood test to check their white cell count, and possibly for a change of working environment.

RADIOACTIVE ISOTOPES

These are substances which have been exposed to a powerful source of atomic energy. Consequently they have become radioactive themselves, without any alteration occurring in their chemical properties. Radioactive isotopes have been found to have a place in the treatment of carcinomas, where the radioactivity destroys malignant cells and hence shrinks tumours. Commonly used isotopes are caesium 137, radium and cobalt 60. They can be applied in one of two ways; either implanted in a cavity, as in the case of carcinoma of the cervix or uterus, or implanted interstitially, in the form of needles, as in carcinoma of the tongue.

Sometimes patients come to theatres to have applicators fitted, into which the radioactive isotope will later be loaded in the x-ray department. Sometimes however, the isotope itself is placed in situ in the operating theatre. The health risks to staff are the same as those associated with x-rays, but it must be remembered that the isotopes are a far more potent source of irradiation as they are constantly emitting rays, with a cumulative effect upon health.

If an isotope is to be introduced in theatre, these are some of the safety measures which must be taken. The theatre used should be well away from the mainstream of department traffic, and again minimal staff should be involved. Certainly no pregnant women should be present. Clear warning signs that there is a radiation hazard must be displayed outside the theatre, so that no one will enter accidentally. The staff involved must all wear radiation detection badges. Lead coats offer no protection against radioactive isotopes as they do against x-rays. The former are a far more potent source of gamma irradiation.

The isotope must be kept inside a lead container. It is delivered to the department in a container which is unsterile, and transferred to a sterile lead container for the operative procedure. The trolley on to which it is transferred should have the added protection of a lead screen. Long handling forceps are used to move the isotope; it should never be touched with the bare hands.

Once all the equipment is assembled, the best protection for staff is to keep their distance while the surgeon operates as quickly as possible. Speed and distance should keep radiation exposure levels to a minimum. To double the distance between oneself and a radioactive source is to reduce the intensity of one's exposure to a quarter of the initial exposure. To treble that distance reduces the exposure to a ninth of the initial exposure, and so on, governed by the inverse square law.

To protect the healthy tissue of the patient, an x-ray is often performed in theatre to check the correct positioning of the implant. The isotopes destroy the healthy cells which they come into contact with as well as malignant ones. To protect other patients in the department, patients with radioactive implants should be nursed in an isolated corner of recovery.

Careful records are kept in the operating department of all isotopes which enter and leave, along with the relevant patient details. This is because radioactive isotopes are not only dangerous, but also very expensive. Any losses must be immediately reported to the radiation protection officer.

LASERS

Some hospitals, usually the more affluent ones, have lasers for use in the treatment of carcinomas. They are most commonly found in the ENT theatre, where they are effective in the treatment of carcinoma of the larynx. They are highly accurate, with the ability to isolate and destroy individual malignant cells. This makes them particularly successful in dealing with the early stages of a new growth. Like radioactive isotopes, the laser beam will also destroy any healthy tissue with which it comes into contact. There is a particular danger to the eyes of staff. When the laser is in use, all staff present should wear protective plastic goggles and avoid looking directly at the beam. Warning signs must again be displayed outside the theatre.

The other hazard posed by lasers is that since they are so very expensive, they constitute a security hazard. Care must be taken to ensure their safe storage.

ANAESTHETIC GASES

Most operating departments now have effective scavenging systems to remove from the atmosphere anaesthetic gases exhaled by patients. Thus the risks associated with a build-up of inflammable waste are also removed, and the effect of the gases on staff health is greatly reduced. You may still be affected initially however, finding yourself unusually tired after work. This is due to small amounts of gas inhaled throughout the day, with nitrous oxide being the main culprit.

It has been suggested in recent years that prolonged exposure to anaesthetic gases can have other, more sinister side-effects. Links have been suggested with decreased fertility and a higher than average spontaneous abortion rate amongst female staff. Nothing has been proven conclusively, but if you are planning a career in the department and also planning to try for a family at some time, it is something to bear in mind. It is probably best to avoid spending the first 3 months of pregnancy working in the department.

BLOOD CONTAMINATION

It is worth mentioning again that all blood spillages should be treated with great care. Always wear gloves if you are mopping up blood or handling bloody equipment, and be sure to use the correct cleaning solutions prescribed by your department. Sharps should similarly be handled with caution, taking care to ensure their correct and safe disposal. Any cuts sustained from handling used sharps, no matter how small, should be reported to the nursing officer and an accident form completed. All blood is a potential infective agent, and blood-borne diseases are not always diagnosed preoperatively.

These are the major environmental health hazards in the operating department. Remember that it is *your* responsibility to take reasonable care of yourself and your colleagues. This means finding out what the hazards are, and the correct, safe working methods which will minimize their effects. Ask trained staff about any unfamiliar equipment, and don't try to operate any until the safe method of doing so has been demonstrated to you.

As well as understanding the source of potential hazards, you should also understand your own physical response to the department, in terms of its effect upon your health. Some symptoms of physical stress you will have encountered in other areas of health care, but some are peculiar to the operating department. These are some of the commonest complaints, and ways in which you might alleviate them.

FAINTING AND PROLONGED STANDING

It is fairly common for staff to faint in the operating theatre. Often this is the one humiliation feared by students before they come to work in the department. It is not the sight of blood, as most people think, however, which causes them to faint, but more usually standing, concentrating in one position for a long time, coupled with a low blood sugar. The classical example is the medical student who has skipped breakfast, rushed to theatre to assist with the first case on the list, and who has been standing scrubbed up holding a retractor for a long time.

The best way to avoid fainting is to ensure a good blood sugar level at all times. Breakfast is extremely important, and you should eat well during meal breaks. It is not a good idea to begin that crash diet you have been promising yourself when you come to work in the operating department! The temperature of the theatre, if it is high, may also induce fainting, so adjust the thermostat as necessary for a comfortable working atmosphere. Electric fans can be employed to cool down the scrub team, but only if the surgeon allows this. (Some object to the use of fans, arguing that they distribute dust and bacteria over the wound.)

Should you feel faint at any time, just walk away from the operation and sit down with your head between your knees, breathing deeply. This applies even if you are scrubbed up. Go as soon as you start to feel dizzy and lightheaded; don't wait until you do faint. Everyone will understand and no one will think you a fool. Most senior surgeons and theatre nurses have fainted themselves at some time. If you wait until you faint at the table, you may contaminate the wound as you fall and you run the risk of seriously hurting yourself on the hard floor. Someone else can always take over from you.

If you witness someone else turning very pale and getting that fixed, glazed expression, the precursors to fainting, lead them away from the table immediately and get them to sit as described. If they have already fainted, you can revive them by placing a pillow under their head and elevating their legs. They will soon come round. A cold, wet cloth on the face is also a good stimulant. As soon as they have sufficiently recovered, take them to the rest room and make them have a drink and something to eat.

Prolonged standing, even if you don't faint, can be uncomfortable enough in itself, especially if you have a tendency to varicose veins. Light-weight support tights can be a great help for women, and lying down for 10 minutes with legs elevated when you come off duty works wonders. During a very long operation it is always acceptable for the circulating assistants to sit down. Occasionally, the scrub nurse may also sit, if there are periods when there is not much to do. This is always subject to the surgeon's agreement, of course, and the stool where the scrub nurse sits must be covered with a sterile green towel, so as not to contaminate the back of his or her gown. This is unusual however; the scrub nurse is usually far too busy assisting to be able to sit down. If you find yourself scrubbed up for what is turning out to be a very long operation, do some unobtrusive feet and leg exercises. This helps to stimulate the circulation and temporarily re-distributes the body weight.

BACK PROBLEMS

An aching back goes with aching legs from prolonged standing. If you have had any problems with your back in the past, you should take extra care of yourself in the operating department. As well as a lot of standing, there is also a lot of moving of heavy equipment and lifting patients. If you have inside-theatre porters in the department, have them do the heavy lifting and moving. If not, and you are female, make use of the many men available. There is no reason why male surgeons, anaesthetists and medical students should not wait behind to lift the patient they have just operated on. If there really is no one else available, female staff should share the burden of the patient's weight between four, each taking one lifting pole.

Strain on the back can further be lessened by ensuring that the trolley on to which the patient is to be lifted is at the same height as the operating table, and that all the brakes are on. As on the wards, when lifting a patient in bed, let the quadriceps muscles do the work and keep your back straight.

Above all, be sensible, and don't suffer in silence. If you know that you are putting your back at risk, then say so and insist on getting help.

THIRST

You will probably find that you are unusually thirsty in the operating department. This is due to the intense ventilation, which makes the atmosphere very dry. To compensate for this, you will notice that early staff have a compulsory tea break in the afternoons, while on the wards this is optional, at the discretion of the nurse in charge. Make sure you drink plenty.

It is also a good idea to get right out of the department at lunchtime, preferably into the fresh air. This will help diminish the feelings of claustrophobia often experienced by students in the department, especially those working in suites without any windows. Most departments allow changing time on top of the meal break.

TIREDNESS

Two reasons why you may feel more tired than usual have already been mentioned – the effect of nitrous oxide and a lot of standing. But you are probably also feeling very tired because you have been given an absolute barrage of new ideas and information about this strange, unusually confined department. Make allowances for yourself. One positive aspect of operating department nursing is its off-duty. This tends to be far more attractive than the rotas you are used to on the wards. You will probably find that you have a much higher proportion of weekends off and fewer late shifts. So make good use of your weekends and evenings, and catch up on the rest you need.

SKIN AND HAIR

You may find that your skin and hair suffer while you work in the operating department. Wearing masks all day can aggravate spots, and theatre hats tend to make your hair more greasy and very flat at the end of the day. Unfortunately this is one occupational hazard you will have to contend with.

STRESS

As well as these physical stresses, you will no doubt also feel some degree of mental stress. This is inevitable in such a new environment, and it is important to recognize this. You will probably feel disoriented and uncertain of your new role; you may have difficulties relating to your new colleagues or anxieties about patient care. Pressures from your home and personal life can also overspill to colour your attitudes to a new working environment. Don't suppress any of these feelings, but do find someone appropriate to talk to. It may be that letting off steam with your flatmates is enough to make you feel better and reassured. If it is not, and you feel the main problem is peculiar to the nature of operating department work, you should approach one of the trained staff. It is probably best to see whoever has particular responsibility for you, be that a clinical teacher or the sister or staff nurse you work with most. If your anxiety is of a more general nature, not particularly related to the department, you may prefer to see your personal tutor, a colleague from another area or a nurse counsellor. The suggested reading matter at the end of this chapter may also help. Allowing stressful situations to persist will not do you any good. You will not function well in your job, to the detriment of patients and yourself, and your health will eventually be undermined.

While recognizing the stresses to which you are subject, it is also important to have an insight into those experienced by the trained nurses in the department. This is not seeking to excuse any bad behaviour, but to underline the undeniable fact that theatre nursing, while being a satisfying and rewarding career, is also a stressful one. If you have some understanding of their major preoccupations and are in sympathy with their aims, it will help you to function within the department and prevent you from taking offence where none was intended.

The job of the theatre nurse is made up of many strands. Patient safety is the first priority, and you will have observed them planning and delivering care to patients at the most vulnerable point of their entire hospital stay. Their actions often have immediate effects upon the condition of patients, so that their responses to situations, especially emergencies, need to be quick. Commands which may sound very abrupt, even rude, to you, are usually made out of necessity for the safety of patients or staff. Emergencies have to be dealt with there and then; there isn't always time to explain the need for some actions. Be aware of this, and choose your moment later in the day, after the crisis has passed, if you would like an explanation of events. Theatre nurses often appear to student nurses to be obsessive about details of care, and not aware of the individuality of patients at all. Their obsession with what appears to be a minor detail is usually well justified. They have probably had experience of what happens when these details are missed – patients suffering diathermy burns from incorrectly applied diathermy plates or developing pressure sores from lack of thought in positioning. Theatre nurses are obsessive about the safety of their patients.

The pace of work can also be rapid. It is possible for the nurse who is running the list to be totally absorbed in organizing staff and sending for patients to ensure no time-wasting. Time is money, and the need to be cost-effective affects all nurses these days. So even though you may be seeing that this particular nurse is scarcely involved in the operation, he or she is by no means neglecting duty or being lazy.

A chronic shortage of nurses in the operating department has been a feature of everyday life for most theatre nurses in recent years. Those who have stayed in the job are usually highly motivated and enthusiastic, but you will no doubt notice that there are times when they are very tired and pushed to their limits. Many theatre nurses regularly do overtime and on-call duties to cover for shortages. This means that not only do staff work extremely hard, but there is also little opportunity for them to be released for study days and training courses. Bearing this in mind, you will appreciate that a high turnover of students in the department, who need teaching and supervising, puts heavy demands on the regular staff.

Co-ordinating the work of a multidisciplinary team demands diplomacy and good communication skills. The acquisition and practice of such skills is a very complex and demanding business. So many people have to agree on and be kept informed of information affecting the smooth running of an operating list. Acting as co-ordinator creates high levels of stress and friction for the theatre nurses.

Apart from running the lists, there is also a great deal of behind-the-scenes work done, of which you are probably unaware. Equipment has to be maintained and ordered from manufacturers to keep up stock levels. Operations can only be done when the right equipment is available, so meeting deadlines with orders and repairs can be another stressor. Accountability, not only for theatre nurses' own work, but also for the learners they supervise, is yet another. It must be repeated that none of this seeks to excuse any bad behaviour on the part of theatre nurses, but to explain the influences affecting them every day. Sensitivity to their needs will help you to help them, and ultimately benefit the patients.

ETHICAL DILEMMAS

You may find that to be present at certain operations is distressing, either because you find the procedure repugnant or it is in conflict with your religious beliefs. Termination of pregnancy, organ transplantation, especially where a live, healthy donor is involved, and some research programmes commonly affect people in this way. If you do not wish to be present when any of these are in progress, you have every right not to be. Tell the nurse running the list as early as possible about your feelings, and it will be arranged for you to be allocated elsewhere. Your wishes in these circumstances will always be respected.

ACCIDENT FORMS

If you or your colleagues suffer any kind of accident, a form must be completed. This must be stressed yet again. Nothing is too trivial to be reported. If as a result of the accident, disease or injury ensues which affects your ability to work and therefore to maintain your independence, the accident form will protect you. It proves that the accident occurred at work and as a result of conditions at work, and that therefore you have a legal right to compensation from your employer.

Further reading

American Society of Anesthesiologists (1974). Report of an ad hoc committee on the effect of trace anaesthetics on the health of operating room personnel. *Anesthesiology,* **35**, 348.

Astbury C. (1988). *Stress in Theatre Nursing.* RCN Research Series. Middlesex: Scutari Press.

Bond M. (1986). *Stress and Self-awareness: A Guide for Nurses.* London: Heinemann Nursing.

Bunch P. (1986). Beaming in on ENT. *Nursing Times,* **82** (40), pp. 67–8.

Davies A. (1986). Diary of an anxious student. *Nursing Times,* **82** (24), pp. 36–7.

Dixon E. (1986). Ethical dilemmas in surgical nursing. *NAT News,* **23** (6), pp. 16–17

Gillespie C., Gillespie V. (1986). Reading the danger signs. Nursing Times, **82** (31), pp. 24–7.

National Association of Theatre Nurses (1981). *Codes of Practice.* Yorkshire: NATN.

14

Getting the most from your theatre allocation

Whether or not you plan to spend time in the operating department as a trained nurse, there is much to be learnt here which can be positively applied in other areas of health care. It is helpful to analyse what is most beneficial so that you can be more aware of what you might gain from the department, even if you feel that theatre nursing isn't for you. Greater awareness of these assets will help you to *set personal goals*. In this way, even if you do not particularly enjoy your allocation, you will come away with specific experiences and skills, and certainly not feel empy-handed.

On the subject of motivation, remember that an interested, alert and assertive student will always fare better than one who appears uninterested, unresponsive and withdrawn. Decide what it is you want to learn, and then ask questions and demand time to practise until you have understood and are competent to carry out that which most interests you. Trained staff will find you a stimulating challenge and a pleasure to teach.

ANAESTHETIC AND RECOVERY SKILLS

To work in anaesthetics and recovery is to care for patients who are extremely vulnerable. General anaesthetics render them unconscious and completely dependent on staff to see to their bodily movements. The expeience will teach you *how to care for the unconscious patient*; how to prevent the formation of pressure sores, how to position the body so as to preserve intact all nerve tissue and how to move the body without straining or damaging joints. You will be making and recording observations of bodily functions frequently, building up an accurate picture of a patient's vital signs. This is invaluable experience for, as you know, unconscious patients present in many departments: in casualty, on both medical and surgical wards, and in the intensive care unit. The principles of care you will learn in anaesthetics and recovery are widely applicable.

Perhaps the most important skill you will learn from caring for unconscious patients is *care of the airway*. You will learn how to keep it clear and thereby maintain its function when patients have lost their coughing and swallowing reflexes. Learning the *intubation procedure* is an extension of this. In anaesthetics you become familiar with the equipment, the appropriate sizes and the order in which they are required. You learn how it all connects to create an anaesthetic circuit, and how to maintain and check the equipment for safe functioning. All of this becomes second nature. This is invaluable since the same equipment crops up in the emergency box of every department in the hospital. Clearing the airway and intubating patients are the first steps taken when dealing with a respiratory or cardiac arrest. These emergencies are often a great source of anxiety to nursing staff, so a good working knowledge of intubation equipment and the procedure will go a long way towards boosting your confidence in your ability to perform well in an emergency.

Indeed, because of the vulnerability of the patients here, you may even witness an *emergency situation* in anaesthetics or recovery. A patient's airway may need to be rapidly cleared, cardiac output may need to be restored or the effects of primary postoperative haemorrhage may need to be dealt with. In this controlled atmosphere, where a lot of senior staff are available, you can observe the fast, competent responses of others to these situations. You may have the opportunity to help, and thus the chance to examine your own feelings and responses to the situation.

By the end of your allocation you will certainly be more confident in handling a variety of *other equipment and procedures*, due to the relatively high concentration of machinery and technology here. Intravenous infusions and blood transfusions are set up and administered more frequently than on the wards. Suction apparatus and oxygen therapy are also more often used. Monitoring equipment, including sphygmomanometers, ECG electrodes and leads, temperature probes, central venous and arterial pressure monitoring lines will become more familiar. You may have more opportunity to practise catheterization than you have had previously. Knowledge of the use and functioning of the anaesthetic machine and cylinders is also very valuable. Theatres are not the only place where they are found. You may well come across them in casualty, the intensive care unit and perhaps also in midwifery.

A general insight into the principles of anaesthesia, both general and local, and a knowledge of the drugs commonly used and their side-effects will stand you in good stead. We have already noted that anaesthetics is a growing specialty: witness the fact that anaesthetists run intensive care units and pain control clinics, as well as having other commitments throughout the hospital, such as giving epidurals on the labour ward. Wherever you choose to work eventually, you will no doubt draw on the knowledge gained during this allocation from time to time.

PATIENT PREPARATION

The biggest single overall gain to be made from the operating department experience is the vast improvement in your ability to prepare patients for surgery. You can now share with greater confidence your increased knowledge of surgery with both patients and their families, and gain greater credence from both. You can offer greater *psychological support*. What you learnt during pre- and postoperative visits and when caring for conscious patients in the department will certainly have tested and stretched your powers of reassurance. You can allay patients' fears about the anaesthetic room, for example. You can tell them what it looks, sounds and smells like; who will be there and what will happen to them. You can explain what they will be asked to do. With regard to surgery, you are now in a much better position to describe operative procedures, types of incisions, and give more realistic time estimates for operations. You will know if a patient is likely to have an intravenous infusion or drainage device postoperatively, and what kind of dressing will be applied. (I once nursed a lady who was convinced that she had had a mastectomy instead of a breast lump biopsy, because no one had explained to her that she might have a bulky pressure dressing postoperatively!) From having witnessed the amount of tissue trauma that can occur during surgery, you will appreciate that patients need to expect to feel pain. (You will also be more aware of the need to relieve it.) You can explain to patients that they will spend some time in recovery, and that it is normal to feel nausea as well as pain.

You are in a much better position to confront patients' fears. You know what the department is like; you have been there and seen what goes on. So give your patients the benefit of your experience, and don't miss out the important details. If you felt afraid in the department initially, just try to imagine how your patients are feeling. It is valuable to keep this memory alive.

Working in the department will also have given you a more sound understanding of preoperative measures taken in the *physical preparation* of patients for surgery. You now know why patients have to be nil by mouth and why their dentures have to be removed; you have seen the intubation procedure. You understand why it is important to clean and mark the skin at the site of operation, why jewellery is removed and an operation gown put on. You understand the need for clean bedding, for completing a preoperative check list and recording a patient's weight and any allergies. You appreciate the need for good timing in giving premedications, and for checking that the patient leaves the ward with a complete set of notes and x-rays. All of this makes complete sense now. Having witnessed how the care delivered in the operating department requires all of the above needs to be satisfied if the patient is to have a safe and smooth passage through theatre, you will not now forget their significance. You can communicate your knowledge to your patients and their families, and advise how their physical condition can be improved preoperatively, for example by giving up smoking or losing weight.

As well as giving an improved service to your patients, you also have *more to offer colleagues* – be they theatre nurses, ward nurses, medical staff and any juniors whom you supervise. You now have a complete overall picture of how they all participate in the care of patients; what their peculiar needs, concerns and potential problems are. Experience gained in the operating department will help you to see your role in this overall scheme of things, whichever aspect of surgical nursing you choose to pursue eventually.

SURGICAL EXPERIENCE AND SKILLS

In the operating theatre you will see the *anatomy*, both normal and abnormal, demonstrated as never before. Seeing the bodily structures and organs, their size, colour and texture, and how they all inter-relate is something of a revelation in itself. You soon realize that flat textbook illustrations and distorted, discoloured specimens immersed in preservative, from which you are used to learning, bear only a scant resemblance to the real thing.

Working as a scrub nurse will have taught you a certain amount of *manual dexterity*, in that you will have learnt to pass instruments swiftly, and in such a manner that they can be used immediately. It will also have taught you more about *asepsis*, where the principles learnt on the wards are practised more scrupulously and thoroughly. Not only will this benefit your own dressing technique, but it will make you a more confident and able assistant to medical staff carrying out sterile procedures in other areas. Your knowledge of surgical nursing will also encompass a greater understanding of the process of *wound healing*, the use of suture materials, drainage devices and what types of dressings are suitable for which wounds.

One very attractive aspect of working in the operating department is that you will find yourself in the midst of a very high concentration of trained staff. This usually releases you from being the main workforce, as on the wards, allowing you more freedom and time to be a real student. You have the opportunity to observe different approaches to management. Use the theatre nurses as role models, observing how they put their clinical judgement into action, and assessing their interpersonal skills. Try to be aware of the amount of planning they put into their day, and try to judge how effective they are. Above all, these are very senior nurses with a wealth of experience between them, so use them as a valuable knowledge source.

There is also a high concentration of medical staff constantly working in the department. The team effort of care delivered to patients will be more obvious to you, and in order for this to happen, you will find yourself having to communicate with them more frequently than is necessary in many other areas. The operating department offers the opportunity to gain more confidence in dealing with medical staff, discussing patients' requirements and jointly putting these into action.

Learning to keep accurate and complete records of care, and appreciating the need for doing so, is something else you will gain in the operating department. Theatre nurses are more attuned to the requirements of the law. Due to the vulnerability of the patients for whom they care, they have a greater potential to commit acts of negligence where the results can be serious or even fatal. This does not mean that they are more negligent than other nurses, but that errors made when a patient is anaesthetized and has an open abdomen, for instance, have a greater potential to harm the patient than those made by ward nurses, when a patient is fully conscious and intact. This difference accounts for the fact that a comparatively larger number of theatre nurses become involved in litigation. Once qualified you will be accountable for the care you give, so the habit of meticulous record keeping is a good one to acquire. If the state of affairs in the USA is one which we will inherit, it is essential that you become aware of your own liabilities and legal issues surrounding your work. Accurate records demonstrating competent care will be your best defence.

These are some suggestions of how there is much to be gained from your operating department allocation. You may well be able to think of other valuable assets the department possesses. The point of highlighting these areas is to set you thinking about how to make the best use of your time here, and to suggest that even if you feel you have no affinity for theatre nursing, there are still many personal gains to be made. Decide what it is you want to learn, and view the allocation from that angle – as a means of satisfying personal goals.

Having set your goals, you need to attain them. Asking questions may not always be enough. Some skills need to be practised under supervision, and even better, assessed. The best way to ensure that you receive feedback on your personal and professional development, where busy staff are notoriously forgetful about constructive criticism, is to collar a trained member of staff, and get them to assess you on one particular procedure, e.g. assisting with an intubation or acting as a circulator or scrub nurse for an operation. This is relatively painless and good for them. It forces them to be more analytical, and is invaluable for you. Better still, get them to commit themselves to paper, so that you have a written record of your progress. Through discussion of their comments, you can jointly decide where improvements can be made. Assessment or report forms provided by the School of Nursing may be adequate for this purpose; if not, why not carry a notebook of your own to use?

Knowing in advance what you want to learn can help shape your allocation. If you would particularly like to be placed in one area or one theatre, why not ask? It is usually possible to accommodate such wishes. When there are quiet periods in your area, you can ask to be released to see what is happening elsewhere in the department. Why not ask the trained staff or your clinical teacher for sessions on particular subjects that interest you? This is usually welcomed. These suggestions are of particular use if you are approaching your finals, and therefore not so ready to absorb a lot of new information, but needing to revise already familiar topics. The range of surgical specialties practised within the operating department makes it an advantageous place to be at this time in your career.

Take the initiative. Get the most out of your theatre allocation, and come away with knowledge and new skills which will enrich your contribution to society as a trained nurse.

15

Operating department nursing as a career

IS IT NURSING?

There has always been a general feeling in the profession that working in the operating department is not really part of nursing. Those who have chosen it as a career have in some way opted out of the mainstream. They have chosen to become task-oriented technicians in a department isolated from the rest of the hospital, hiding from patients. As long as such a feeling exists it is little wonder that you may feel dubious about your operating department allocation. The record needs to be put straight.

Are the major concerns and functions of theatre nurses so very different from those of nurses in other departments? Theatre nurses would dispute this. Let us consider this in the light of a recent definition of nursing. At the Geneva International Council of Nurses in 1979, it was stated that the prime function of nursing was 'to assist the individual, sick or well, in the performance of those activities contributing to health or its recovery (or to a peaceful death) that he should perform unaided if he had the necessary strength, will or knowledge'. (Henderson, 1979).

From what you have read so far, and the experience you gain in the operating department, it will be clear that a high standard of care and service to patients is the theatre nurse's top priority. This incorporates both psychological and physical care. The introduction of the nursing process in many departments reflects this, demonstrating that the concern of theatre nurses for contributing to individualized patient care ranks alongside that of ward nurses. As theatre nurses now regularly leave the department to visit patients both pre- and postoperatively, they can no longer be accused of being isolated or impersonal. Nor are they lacking in compassion. They share with patients and their relatives their knowledge and experience. They share with surgical nurses the common aims of promoting good health and a smooth, uneventful recovery from surgery.

Indeed the role of the theatre nurse is crucial to these aims. They are caring for patients undergoing anaesthesia, surgery and immediately postoperatively; the stages of care for which purpose the hospital admission was arranged. At this time patients are at their most dependent and most vulnerable, so the theatre nurse's care has a greater potential to affect a successful outcome to surgery and a subsequent return to normal living. It should also be remembered that theatre nurses have the ideal opportunity to deliver high standards of nursing care. They deal with one patient at a time, so that patients receive their full attention, instead of competing with 24 others, as in a ward situation. Patient care is the first priority of theatre nurses, and one which they can practise very successfully. Is this hiding away from patients?

If service to patients is the prime concern of theatre nurses, care of colleagues and their environment ranks a close second. They care about the general welfare, health, education, personal and professional development of their colleagues. They try to ensure that their department is safe for everyone to work in, that its stress potential is kept to a minimum and that it functions smoothly and cost-effectively. What is the difference so far between this and the mainstream of nursing?

There is some truth in the fact that the department is geographically and atmospherically removed from the rest of the hospital but, as explained in Chapter 2, this is necessary to minimize the possible introduction of harmful bacteria. Operating departments rely on the back-up services of a vast array of others however, and you will notice a constant stream of visitors. So it is not strictly true to say that theatre nurses are isolated; indeed they enjoy participating in teamwork of a truly multidisciplinary nature.

With such a high emphasis on patients first, theatre nurses do not have time these days to be task-oriented – another false accusation. In the past, well yes, they might have been more so, but they are now backed up by a full range of support services – domestics, porters, receptionists and TSSU staff.

Are they just mechanics? No, this is also not true. They may have to deal with more machinery than a ward nurse, but not more than a nurse who works in the intensive care unit, or indeed a midwife. ODAs have gradually assumed more and more responsibility for this aspect of the department's work. In 1984, when they came under the auspices of the Professional and

Technical Council, ODAs expressed the wish to be seen not as a profession challenging the role of the theatre nurse, but as one with a separate, complementary identity. The objectives of the Lewin Report (1970), London: HMSO, appear to have finally been achieved in the 1980s. Nurses and ODAs now coexist happily within the department, without the fear that each is trying to impinge upon the role of the other. It has been conceded beyond doubt that there is a place and need for professional nurses within the operating department. Who else should be responsible for the care of patients during the most stressful and vulnerable period of their entire hospital stay? Would nurses not be betraying their ideals and patients' trust if they were to abandon them outside the department's doors? Theatre nurses as senior theatre managers have similarly demonstrated their worth over the years. With only a few exceptions throughout the country, they still occupy these positions of responsibility.

So there are no grounds for saying that theatre nurses do not belong truly to the rest of the nursing profession. There is no difference between their concerns and preoccupations and those of nurses in other areas. It could be argued that it is part of nursing and much more! More immediately influenced by advancing technology, the greater sophistication in surgical and anaesthetic techniques is constantly reflected in theatre nursing skills, endowing it with the potential to become infinitely more exciting in the future. Time has shown that theatre nurses are able to respond to and absorb such changes, while leaving intact the fundamental commitment to service to patients and colleagues.

WHY OTHERS HAVE CHOSEN IT AS A CAREER

When a cross-section of different ranks of theatre nurses from a variety of both old and new hospitals throughout England and Scotland were interviewed about their choice of career, many different aspects of the job were cited as reasons for their choice (Cain, 1985). One common factor was that they had all enjoyed their student allocation to the department, and felt that they had gained a lot from it.

The most attractive aspect of the job, most frequently mentioned, was that it encompasses much variety, and therefore keeps theatre nurses in touch with a broad spectrum of specialties. The nurses felt able to function competently and happily in a variety of different environments throughout the hospital. Coping with emergencies in the operating department gave them the confidence that they would be able to cope well with an emergency arising elsewhere. All of these factors had the positive spin-off of opening many doors to them when they felt it was time to move on and work in other departments.

Many felt that working in theatres either complemented or provided an interesting contrast to other nursing experiences. Those who had worked on surgical wards since qualification particularly felt this. Working in theatres had greatly improved their skills as surgical nurses, bringing many of the benefits discussed in Chapter 14, and much more excitement. Midwives who opted to work in theatres reported that being able to scrub up and assist with caesarean sections added the finishing touch to their midwifery training.

Indeed, enjoyment of the drama element in theatres attracted many staff back to work there. This was generated by the need to respond immediately to situations – thinking quickly and solving problems on their feet. Theatre nurses enjoyed this challenge, especially when related to on-call duties. Some mentioned that they enjoyed nothing better than being called out in the middle of the night, when staff are few, and when their thorough knowledge of their job was really appreciated.

Problem-solving, in relation to applying nursing knowledge and skills imaginatively, not necessarily in an emergency, was also a great source of satisfaction. Theatre nurses felt that they could apply anatomy and physiology here more than in other areas, particularly when positioning patients for surgery and in selecting the appropriate equipment and instruments. These kinds of comments were made more frequently by nurses working in specialist fields, particularly in cardiac and neurosurgery.

With the constant introduction of new equipment and materials, nursing and medical procedures are constantly being up-dated. Theatre nurses found responding to such change very stimulating. They reported never feeling bored or complacent about their knowledge, especially in recent years when advances in technology have been more apparent. Many nurses also mentioned satisfaction from attaining deeper levels of understanding from their work. From a superficial knowledge of what was involved in certain procedures, which allowed them to function adequately initially, many felt that they had in time built on that knowledge considerably, increasing their understanding and ultimately becoming very able surgical assistants. Instead of just having a basic 'recipe' for assisting with surgery – knowing the usual order in which the instruments and sutures are normally required – deeper understanding allowed them the ability to assess more accurately the progress of the operation by being able to interpret what they saw, and to act accordingly.

Having one patient to care for at a time was also a big attraction. Many nurses had left the wards because of intense frustration at not being able to deliver the care patients needed, through lack of time and opportunity. In the operating department this is not a problem; nurses can give care which matches up to their ideals.

Many social reasons were also cited in choosing a career in operating department nursing. Although they visit patients on the wards both pre- and postoperatively, they are not constantly with them and unlike ward nurses they become less emotionally involved with their lives. Those who had had ward experience reported greater peace of mind while working in theatres for this reason. They felt able to go home and forget work more easily, knowing that they had given a high standard of care, but that now the responsibility for patients had been reassumed by the ward nurses. This was a particularly important issue for nurses with family commitments, who felt that once in the home they could give their undivided attention to partners and children, without the added stress of worrying about patients. For these nurses, theatre nursing was also more convenient, as 'cold' surgery takes place between the hours of 9 a.m.–5 p.m. Monday to Friday, and operating departments have traditionally shown a greater willingness to employ part-time staff than other areas. Indeed many nurses, including those without family commitments, mentioned that the attractiveness of theatre's off-duty rota had had an influence upon their career choice. Those who could compare this with other experiences reported that more weekends and evenings off made them feel fresher and more able to be objective about their work.

PLANNING A CAREER IN THE OPERATING DEPARTMENT

If you have enjoyed your time in the department and feel that theatre nursing could be a career possibility for you, it is a good idea to discuss returning to the department at a later date. Speak to your theatre sister, clinical teacher or nursing officer about this. They can advise you about your suitability for the work and in the future, when they are filling job vacancies, they will remember that you were the student who approached them, showing interest and enthusiasm. After you have been back in the department for a further few months as a trained nurse, you will be in a better position to decide whether or not this is the career you want.

If it is, it is best for you to try and get a place on an English National Board course 176. This is not strictly essential, as it is still possible to progress up the hierachy without a course in some hospitals, but the benefits for you are considerable. The course lasts 54 weeks, of which 10 are spent in the School of Nursing; the remaining time rotates through different surgical specialties, anaesthetics and recovery. Four weeks are set aside for you to choose a placement of special interest, and this need not be restricted to the hospital where you are based.

There is a variety of practical experience to be gained, which is simultaneously supported by a high level of theoretical knowledge. Anatomy and physiology are thoroughly revised, which is especially valuable to those who did their basic training some years previously. Lectures are given by all the relevant specialists whose work connects them to the operating department in some way, such as surgeons, the nurse counsellor, the hospital solicitor, safety officers, supplies managers and the TSSU manager, to mention a few. Relevant outside visits are also arranged, perhaps to an instrument or suture manufacturer's, or to another kind of specialist theatre, for example. The course aims to cover all aspects of general surgery, some specialties, and to give an overall insight into the running and maintenance of the operating department. The course is also designed to develop the teaching and managerial skills of the student, and to stimulate interest in further education and professional issues. There is a heavy emphasis on student presentation and problem-solving exercises. Each student undertakes a detailed project during the course, which is presented towards the end, and there is usually also a final written examination. All of this is co-ordinated by a specially appointed course tutor, sometimes also working in conjunction with a clinical teacher.

Apart from the final examination, students are also subject to continuous assessment, both in school and throughout each placement. This is a two-way process however, as students are asked to evaluate the course module by module. This means that the course develops according to the direction of the students, constantly modified to meet their needs. As they are a group of trained nurses on a post-basic education course, the group members have a powerful voice within the department. Any changes for the better advocated by them in procedures or policy are always seriously considered.

There are usually between 4 and 12 students on a course, so plenty of individual attention is guaranteed. Learning as one of a group can be stimulating, and you will undoubtedly learn a lot from your peers. Moving to a new hospital can seem daunting, but it is less so if you know you are going to meet others doing the same thing. Being part of a group gives a sense of identity, of belonging, and a potential nuclear social life in a new environment. So getting a place on an English National Board course has many benefits you would not enjoy if you simply stayed working in the operating department as a staff nurse. You will see operating department nursing in a much wider context, being aware of a broad spectrum of issues surrounding the work and having an insight into related interests. You will have received plenty of feedback and support with regard to your personal and professional development, which will give you the confidence to progress in your career. Above all, it will have been an enjoyable experience, contributing to the development of a learning programme and being stimulated by a peer group.

There is also a specialist English National Board anaesthetics course run at about half a dozen centres throughout Britain. This may be the aspect of operating department nursing which particularly appeals to you. This is a 6-month course.

Once the course is over you should consolidate your experience, for you will find that this is the period when things really begin to fall in place and when you really begin to learn. The short placements of the course are really just tasters of different aspects of the department; you need several months or even years to become really familiar with particular areas. When you have a minimum of 2 years' solid theatre experience behind you, this is usually when you are considered eligible to start applying for junior sister posts. There are no hard and fast rules about this however; it depends on whether you feel ready to shoulder more responsibility, and upon the local policy of the hospitals where you apply.

From a sister, the progression up the nursing hierarchy is much the same as for other nurses. The choices are administration, as a nursing officer, and up through the ranks of senior nurses, or teaching, as a course tutor or clinical teacher. As discussed in Chapter 3, with the publication of the Griffiths Report (see Glossary) which introduced competition from non-nursing personnel to control the purse strings of this relatively large departmental budget, and with increased computerization, this is an exciting time to be in management. One opportunity which does not exist for other nurses is the post of TSSU manager.

As you can appreciate, a theatre nursing qualification is a very valuable one. Theatre nurses are a precious commodity; they will never be short of a job. There are always plenty of theatre vacancies in the NHS, which means that agency work as well as full-time posts is also plentiful. Many agencies will pay a higher hourly rate to qualified theatre nurses, and indeed it is currently under discussion between the profession and the government whether this should not also be the case in the NHS. There are also many posts available in the private sector and abroad. Here there are better remuneration and perks than in the NHS, and often the chance for the ambitious to be more rapidly promoted to theatre manager. Once you have your operating department qualification, the world can still be your oyster, even though this may no longer still be true for general nurses without a specialist skill.

Theatre nurses have their own professional organization, the National Association of Theatre Nurses (NATN), which you can join for an annual subscription. This organization produces a regular journal, *NAT News*, which carries articles on research, management and educational topics. NATN also organizes an annual conference, which has been held in Harrogate in recent years. Each conference has a theme which is discussed from a multitude of angles, and new innovations in surgery and nursing are presented. A huge trade exhibition runs simultaneously, where medical representatives can demonstrate new equipment and theatre nurses can shop around. NATN also has many thriving local branches which meet regularly throughout the year. There is a well oiled professional network available to support theatre nurses, mainly supplied by NATN, but relevant literature is also available through various publishing houses and the Royal College of Nursing. The *Nursing Times and Nursing Mirror* also has an annual theatre nursing supplement to coincide with the

NATN conference.

These are just a few ideas on planning a career in operating department nursing, and some of the benefits you will reap if you do.

References

Cain A. (1985). Constructive criticism. (Theatre Nursing Supplement), *Nursing Mirror*, **161**, pp. 85–8.
Henderson V. (1979). *Basic Principles of Nursing Care*, Geneva: International Council of Nurses.

Further reading

Brett H. Did we stick to the brief? *Nursing Times*, **74**(42), pp. 1717–18.
Donn M. Don't write our requiem. *Nursing Mirror*, **149** (15), pp. ii–v.
Fox J. A. (1985). The battle for supremacy. *Nursing Mirror*, **161**, pp. 82–4.
Girot E. (1985). The end of the line? *Senior Nurse*, **3**, pp. 28–30.
Levy C.J. (1978). ODAs march on. *Nursing Times*, **74** (42), pp. 1716–17.
Lewin W. (1978). The organisation and staffing of operating departments. *Nursing Times*, **74** (42), pp. 1711.
Smith J. An ODA is not a nurse. *Nursing Times*, **74** (42), pp. 1714–15.
Wang D. (1978). Patient care before labels for staff. *Nursing Times*, **74** (42), pp. 1715–16.
Williams M. (1978). Theatre of protest. *Nursing Mirror*, **148** (11), pp. 20–2.

16

Operations you may scrub up for

The aim of this chapter is to try to piece together all the information already discussed. It describes in detail four operations which you may well find yourself scrubbing up for, demonstrating how principles of care are translated into action. It must be remembered that all surgeons differ in their requirements, so that the information regarding sutures, dressings and instruments provide guidelines only. This chapter also takes routine preparation and postoperative care for granted, such as care of the airway after general anaesthetic. Special preparation and postopertaive points are peculiar to that operation only. The descriptions given are not nursing care plans, but summaries of operative procedures.

DILATATION AND CURETTAGE

Description: This is an operation performed by the gynaecological surgeons. Prior to the procedure the bladder is catheterized. (An empty bladder is far less at risk of being traumatized than a full, bulging one.) The cervix is then gripped by two strong clamps, via the vagina, and the os is gradually dilated. This gives the surgeon access to the endometrium – the lining of the uterus. Endometrial tissue can thus be removed using a curette.

Rationale: This operation has therapeutic value in treating menstrual disorders. Removing the top layer of endometrial cells which fail to shed monthly is usually beneficial. It is also carried out for diagnostic purposes, to detect the presence of abnormal tissue, such as carcinomas or polyps.

Special preparation: None.

Anaesthetic: General. A face mask and airway are sufficient as this is only a short procedure, lasting 5–10 minutes.

Position: Lithotomy.

Draping: Lithotomy.

Special instruments required:

Metal catheter.

Speculae: similar to retractors, to give access to the vagina.

Vulsellae: angled, toothed clamps for gripping the cervix.

Uterine sound: a curved instrument with measuring gradations. This is for measuring the size of the uterine cavity and for assessing its shape – whether it is anteverted or retroverted.

Hegar's dilators: a range of slightly curved instruments with a gradually increasing diameter size, used to dilate the cervical os.

Polyp forceps.

Ovum forceps.

Bladder sound.

Curettes.

(No diathermy required.)

Procedure: A waterproof paper sheet is placed under the patient's buttocks.

Perineum and vagina are cleaned.

Draping.

Patient is catheterized. (Sometimes a specimen of urine is required for microbiology, so check with the surgeon before handing out the urine to the circulating nurse.)

Speculum is inserted.

Vulsellae are clamped on to the cervix so that it can be pulled gently forwards.

The uterus is sounded (unless the patient is thought to be pregnant).

Cervical os is dilated.

Endometrial tissue is removed with a curette and collected on a clean swab.

Finally, the vagina is swabbed dry and the instruments removed. A sanitary pad is placed over the vagina.

Specimen: The curettings are carefully handled with non-toothed forceps, so as not to obscure their histology. They are preserved in formol saline in a well labelled pot.

Special postoperative points: Observe for vaginal bleeding. (A rare complication of this procedure is a ruptured uterus.)

EXCISION BIOPSY OF BREAST LUMP

Description: Dissection of a segment of breast tissue.

Rationale: This operation is done purely for diagnostic purposes, to detect the presence of carcinomas of the breast.

Special preparation: These patients obviously need a lot of psychological support. They are afraid that they may have cancer and also worried about the cosmetic results of the operation. They need to be reassured about the limits of the operation, i.e. that the surgeon will not proceed to a mastectomy without their written consent, and should be warned that they will have a bulky pressure dressing in situ postoperatively.
Axilla shave on the affected side.
Medical staff need to locate the lump and clearly mark the skin.

Anaesthetic: Usually general with a face mask and airway. Day patients can also have the procedure performed under local anaesthetic however.

Position: Prone. It may be useful to position the arm away from the side using an arm board, so that the surgeon has better access. Diathermy plate in situ.

Draping: Square method around the breast. A small towel is adequate to cover the patient's head. An extra small towel will be needed for the arm if it is extended on an arm board.

Instruments: Small general set, containing:
Allis tissue forceps.
McIndoe scissors.
Catspaw retractors.
Small Langenbeck retractors.

Procedure: Skin cleaning.
Draping.
Skin is incised with a small blade, usually no. 10.
Adipose tissue is incised using McIndoe scissors, with a small pair of toothed forceps to grip.
Bleeding points are diathermized.
Retractors are inserted to give good access to the lump.
Surgeon grasps the lump with tissue forceps, and dissects it out using scissors and non-toothed forceps.
Diathermy is used to ensure haemostasis before closure.
(The wound is made as small as possible. This is for cosmetic reasons, and to ensure minimal handling and subsequent bruising

of the very vascular breast tissue.)

Specimen: This is placed in a well labelled pot of formol saline. Specimens for frozen section remain dry and are sent immediately to the pathology laboratory.

Sutures: 2/0 plain or chromic catgut on a round-bodied needle for the breast and adipose tissue.
4/0 ethilon on a curved cutting needle for skin.

Dressing: Gauze covered by Elastoplast strapping, which stretches right across the affected side of the chest. Cotton wool or a dressing pad can be added for extra pressure.

Special postoperative points: Psychological support. Never say anything to patients about what the surgeon said of the appearance of the lump. Let medical staff deal with this.
Observe the wound for bruising or haematoma. (Occasionally a Redivac drain may be in situ.)

VASECTOMY

Description: Removing a segment of vas on either side and ligating the cut ends.

Rationale: To arrest the flow of sperm from the testes to the shaft of the penis; a contraceptive operation. (The procedure can be reversed by re-anastomosing the cut ends of vas, but success is not guaranteed. The longer the time gap between the two operations, the slimmer the chances are of success.)

Special preparation: These patients need counselling to enable them to decide whether or not they really want the operation carried out. If this is to be done under local anaesthetic, they need a full explanation of what to expect and a great deal of reassurance because of the embarrassing nature of the operation.
Groin shave if necessary.

Anaesthetic: This can be done under general anaesthetic, using a mask and airway, but is more frequently done under local these days, as most cases are day patients.

Position: Prone. If the patient is awake, he may be more comfortable propped up with a couple of pillows.

Draping: Square, with the scrotum exposed on top of the towels. If a local anaesthetic is being given, remember that an anaesthetic screen should be in situ. Make sure that the patient cannot see the operation, and that his breathing is not inhibited by the extra drapes around the face.

Instruments: Small general set, containing:
Halstead artery forceps.
Allis tissue forceps.
Small curved round-ended scissors (Kilner).
You will need to add syringes, needles and a filling tube if local anaesthetic is to be used.
No diathermy plate should be used.

Procedure: Ensure the comfort of the patient.
Clean the skin (using warmed solutions if the patient is awake).
Drape.
The surgeon identifies the vas at the neck of the scrotum.
Local anaesthetic is injected.
Small skin incision is made using a no. 10 blade, through which the vas is delivered using artery forceps.
The vas is gripped by tissue forceps, and gradually more of its length is delivered through the wound.
Two artery forceps are clamped on to the vas, occluding the lumen, and then two cuts are made using the inside knife, with a no. 15 blade. A length of vas is thus removed (Fig. 16.1).
The two cut ends are then ligated and the artery forceps removed.
The scrotum is sutured in one layer.
The procedure is repeated on the other side.

Specimens: The vas is sent for histology in formol saline, to verify that the surgeon has cut the correct structure.
Ensure that the pots are clearly labelled 'left' and 'right', and that the correct specimen goes into each. (This is important, as should it transpire that it is not vas which has been cut on one side, the surgeon needs to know which side needs further attention. Incorrect labelling could lead to an unnecessary operation and an unwanted pregnancy!)

Sutures: 3/0 plain catgut or dexon ties for the vas.
3/0 or 4/0 chromic catgut or dexon on a curved trocar pointed needle for the scrotum.

Dressing: Usually Opsite spray directly on to the wound, covered by a small piece of gauze and further spray to hold it in place. A scrotal support can help prevent swelling.

Special postoperative points: If the patient is going home directly, it must be explained to him that his sutures will dissolve. He also

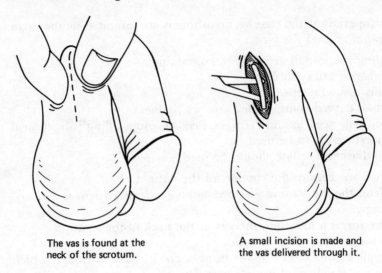

The vas is found at the
neck of the scrotum.

A small incision is made and
the vas delivered through it.

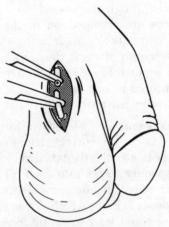

Ligate the ends after removing a
section of vas. Close the scrotum
in a single layer.

Fig. 16.1 Vasectomy procedure

needs to be told to observe the wounds for any further bleeding
or signs of infection. You can reinforce medical advice that no
unprotected intercourse should occur until two successive sperm-
free semen specimens have been obtained.

APPENDICECTOMY

Description: Removal of the appendix via a small incision in the right iliac fossa.

Rationale: This is usually done as an emergency operation on patients with acute appendicitis. If it is not removed, there is a greater danger that the appendix will burst and cause peritonitis. Speed is of the essence.

Special preparation: These patients need a lot of reassurance as they will be in pain, feeling generally very unwell, and because there will be little time between admission and operation. This is especially true if the patient is a child. Remember that the parents will need a lot of support too.
Abdominal shave if necessary.

Anaesthetic: General, using an endotracheal tube. This allows for good abdominal muscle relaxation. Sellick's manoeuvre may need to be employed during intubation if the patient has not starved for long.

Position: Prone. Diathermy plate required.

Draping: Square, around the right iliac fossa.

Instruments: General set, including:
Babcock tissue forceps.
Dunhill artery forceps.
Small and medium Langenbeck retractors.
McIndoe scissors.
Kidney dish for 'dirty' instruments.
Microbiology swab or sterile bottle.

Procedure:
Skin cleaning.
Draping.
Small incision is made over the right iliac fossa using a no. 20 blade. Abdominal muscle is split using the inside knife with a no. 10 blade and toothed dissecting forceps.
Once the muscle is split, the surgeon can free and deliver the appendix on to the outside of the wound, using McIndoe scissors and non-toothed forceps. Langenbeck retractors holding back the muscle edges will facilitate the process.
Diathermy is applied to bleeding vessels as necessary.
Babcock tissue forceps are applied to the bowel for ease of handling.

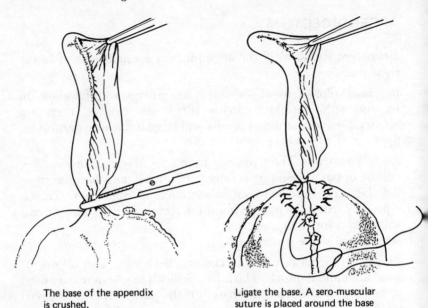

The base of the appendix
is crushed.

Ligate the base. A sero-muscular
suture is placed around the base
of the appendix.

Fig. 16.2   Appendicectomy procedure

Dunhill artery forceps are applied to the mesentery supplying the appendix.

The blood supply is then cut with the scissors, and the ends of vessels ligated.

The appendix stump is crushed between two Dunhills, and the lumen of the bowel is then cut with the inside knife. The specimen and knife are placed in the 'dirty' dish and handed out to the circulator.

A purse-string suture is applied to the base of the appendix, which is then invaginated.

Muscle and skin layers are sutured (Fig. 16.2).

Specimens: The appendix goes into a well labelled pot of formol saline. Microbiology swabs or bottles of pus must go directly to the microbiology department, or else be refrigerated until this is possible, if the operation is performed outside normal working hours.

Sutures: 2/0 chromic catgut ties for the mesentery.

2/0 chromic catgut suture on a round-bodied needle for the pursestring suture on the appendix stump.

2/0 or 0 chromic catgut on a round-bodied needle for the muscle.

(The muscle layer here is relatively thin.)

3/0 ethilon on a straight cutting needle for skin.

Dressing: Airstrip, or Mepore if the patient is allergic to this.

Special postoperative points: Remember to give these patients plenty of reassurance and re-orientation as they wake up.

Glossary

COMMON PREFIXES

Angio: appertaining to blood vessels
Arthro: joints
Cardio: heart
Cholecyst: gallbladder
Colpo: vagina
Cysto: bladder, but can also refer to any fluid-filled sac
Hyster: uterus
Mast: breast
Nephr: kidney
Oophor: ovary
Orchid: testis
Pneum: lung
Pyel: pelvis of kidney
Rhino: nose
Thoraco: chest

COMMON SUFFIXES

desis: a fusion operation, e.g. arthrodesis
ectomy: removal or excision of a structure, e.g. appendicectomy
graphy: representing, recording or describing, e.g. angiography
orrhaphy: repair of a structure, e.g. colporrhaphy
oscopy: looking into the interior of a structure by means of a lighted instrument or endoscope, e.g. cystoscopy
ostomy: constructing an artificial opening into a structure, e.g. colostomy
otomy: incising or dividing a structure, e.g. tenotomy
pexy: suturing or fixing a structure in place, e.g. orchidopexy
plasty: rebuilding or restoring tissues destroyed by disease or injury, e.g. arthroplasty

GLOSSARY OF COMMON TERMS

Abdominoperineal excision of the rectum: where two surgeons work simultaneously to remove the rectum – one via an abdominal incision and the other beginning at the perineum – until the whole of the rectum has been mobilized and removed.

Adhesions: strands of fibrous connective tissue which form between two normally separate structures. They arise out of inflamed or damaged tissue, often as the result of previous surgery.

AIDS: acquired immune deficiency syndrome caused by infection with the HIV virus.

Airway: there are two types of artificial airway. The *oral* type is a short hollow tube that fits into the mouth, anchored by the teeth and lips, and lies on top of the tongue, holding it forwards to maintain a clear passage of air. The *nasopharyngeal* airway is a longer hollow tube performing the same function. It is inserted into the nostril, against which it is anchored in place, keeping a clear air passage to the pharynx.

Anastomosis: creating an artificial communication between two hollow organs, such as blood vessels or sections of bowel.

Aneurysm: a balloon-like swelling in the wall of an artery, due to weakness or sustained damage in its muscular coat. This will eventually burst, and needs urgent surgical repair. A leaking aneurysm constitutes a surgical emergency.

Appendicectomy: removal of the appendix.

Approximation: bringing together two edges until they are in contact, for example, the two skin edges of a wound.

Arteriotomy: an incision into a blood vessel.

Asepsis: the complete absence of bacteria, fungi, viruses or other micro-organisms that could cause infection. The ideal state for surgery. Synonymous with sterility.

Biopsy: Excision of a small piece of tissue for examination.

Caesarean section: delivery of a baby via an incision made in the uterus through the abdomen.

Cardiothoracic: appertaining to the heart and chest.

Cholecystectomy: removal of the gallbladder.

Coagulation: converting liquid blood into a solid state. This is done by means of applying an electrical current, via the diathermy forceps, which seals off bleeding vessels.

Colonoscope: a hollow instrument fitted with a light for inspecting the interior of the colon.

Contaminate: to pollute or infect. Used interchangeably in the text with 'desterilize'.

Cytology: the study of the structure and function of cells.

Defibrillator: a machine for delivering a controlled electric shock to restore normal heart rhythm, where cardiac arrest is due to ventricular fibrillation. The current is delivered via electrodes placed on the chest wall over the heart, or directly on to the heart itself if the chest has been surgically opened.

Desterilize: to render unsterile; bringing a sterile surface into contact with any object which is not sterile.

Detergent: a synthetic cleansing agent that removes impurities from a surface by reacting with grease and tiny suspended particles, including bacteria and other micro-organisms. A detergent is not adequate however for complete disinfection of surfaces.

Diathermy: a high frequency electric current which produces great heat concentration (at the tip of the surgeon's diathermy forceps). It is used to coagulate bleeding vessels or for incising tissue, if the frequency of the current is further increased.

Disinfectant: an agent that destroys or removes bacteria and other micro-organisms, but not necessarily spores. It will therefore not ensure absolute sterility.

ECG: recording of the electrical activity of the heart via electrodes attached to the patient's skin.

Endometrium: the mucous membrane lining the uterus.

Endotracheal tube: a hollow tube reaching from the mouth down to the trachea. Its function is to ensure a clear, controllable airway once the cough reflex has disappeared and the respiratory muscles have been paralysed. It has an inflatable cuff to seal off the lungs from any gastric aspirate.

English National Board courses: post-registration courses in specialist areas of training.

Excision: cutting away or cutting out.

Fibreoptics: synthetic fibres with special optical properties for the transmission of light images. Fibreoptic endoscopes or telescopes containing fibreoptics are in common use, and relay pictures of the inside of the body for direct observation or photography.

French gauge: the Charriere catheter sizes – the circumference in millimetres.

Frozen section: a method of preparing specimens for immediate histological examination. The specimen is frozen into a solid block, instead of being set in wax, the normal method of preparation, which takes much longer. A very thin cross-section can then be cut and viewed under the microscope.

Gauze roll: a length of gauze used for packing cavities postoperatively, e.g. the vagina following vaginal hysterectomy. The gauze has a Raytec thread throughout its entire length.

General manager: administrative post created as a result of the Griffiths Report, 1983 (q.v.) The general manager controls a health district, where 'the responsibility is drawn together in one person, at different levels of organisation, for planning, implementing and control of performance'. The person appointed need not necessarily have any medical background.

Genitourinary surgery: that referring to any part of the urinary system: kidneys, ureters, bladder, urethra and external genitalia.

Griffiths report, 1983: government report on the administration and funding of the NHS under the auspices of Roy Griffiths, a senior official of the successful Sainsburys company. It suggested ways of running the NHS more along the lines of a commercial concern. Probably its most controversial recommendation was the introduction of the general manager.

Haematoma: an accumulation of blood within the tissues that clots to form a solid swelling.

Haemostasis: the state where all bleeding has been arrested.

Hepatitis: inflammation of the liver due to viral infection. Serum hepatitis, is transmitted through contact with infected blood or blood products.

Hernia: the protrusion of an organ or tissue out of the body cavity it normally inhabits, e.g. an inguinal hernia, where a sac of peritoneum containing fat or part of the bowel bulges through the inguinal canal, a weak part of the abdominal wall.

Histology: the study of the structure of tissues by means of special staining techniques combined with light and electron microscopy.

Induction: the initiation of anaesthesia.

Invaginate: to fold in the wall of a solid structure to form a cavity.

Laparoscopy: examination of the abdominal structures, inside the peritoneum, through a hollow lighted instrument.

Laryngoscope: an instrument for examining the larynx. It has a curved blunt metal blade that presses the tongue out of the line of vision and is fitted with a light bulb.

Laryngospasm: closure of the larynx and subsequent obstruction of the air flow to the lungs, usually as part of an allergic reaction.

Ligate: to tie off a bleeding blood vessel or the base of a structure to be excised.

Litigation: the bringing of a lawsuit.

Lumbar sympathectomy: partial excision of sympathetic nervous tissue in the lumbar region, to enhance blood flow to the lower limbs.

Mastectomy: removal of the breast.

Mayo table: a small table on wheels and with an adjustable height; useful in major surgery as a surface on which the scrub nurse can keep only the instruments currently in use. It is usually in position at the bottom of the table, across the patient's feet.

Microsurgery: surgery carried out with the aid of a microscope, hence everything is on a very small, fine scale. Much neurosurgery, middle ear surgery and ophthalmics is microsurgery.

Mitosis: a type of cell division in which a single cell produces two genetically identical daughter cells. This is the way in which new body cells are produced for both growth and repair.

NATN: the National Association of Theatre Nurses, whose headquarters are in Harrogate, North Yorkshire.

Neurosurgery: the surgical treatment of diseases of the brain and spinal cord.

Peroperative cholangiogram: x-ray examination of the common bile duct carried out during cholecystectomy to ensure the removal of all stones. A radiopaque dye is injected directly into the common bile duct and x-rays are taken while the patient is on the table.

Premedication: drugs administered preoperatively to calm and sedate the patient; usually combined with atropine to dry up saliva which might be inhaled under anaesthesia.

Renal calculi: kidney stones, commonly composed of calcium oxalate.

Resection: surgical removal of a part of the body: cutting out or cutting away.

Resistant *Staphylococcus aureus*: a strain of this bacteria, commonly found on the skin and mucous membranes, which does not respond to any antibiotic therapy.

Retropubic prostatectomy: a largely obsolete operation these days, where the prostate gland is removed via an abdominal incision through the prostate capsule.

Ruptured uterus: perforation of the uterus, normally due to instrumentation. This needs urgent repair as the patient will haemorrhage.

Sinus: an infected tract leading from a focus of infection to the surface of the skin or to a hollow organ.

Sling: a narrow length of soft plastic used for retracting and isolating delicate structures, such as blood vessels.

'Splash' bowl: a bowl of water or saline in which surgeons can rinse their gloves.

Staging laparotomy: an operation to assess the progress or stage reached by lymphomas or Hodgkin's disease. The abdomen is opened and multiple biopsies are taken of the liver and lymphatics.

Static electricity: electrical charges at rest, i.e. not flowing in a current.

Sterile field: the entire area covered by sterile surfaces. In the context of an operation, this will be the area covered by sterile green drapes and gowns and the prepared skin of the patient – all the patient's drapes, the trolleys and the scrubbed personnel.

Sterility: the complete absence of any infective material.

Stripping and ligation of varicose veins: the removal of a length of vein containing varicosities by means of a long wire stripper, threaded down the length, and then pulled out at the bottom end. The head attached to the stripper removes the vein as it travels down the inside of the leg. The vein is tied off at the top and bottom.

Transurethrally: access through the urethra. This is the way the prostate gland is commonly removed today, using a resecto-scope, so that no external incision is necessary.

Vaginal hysterectomy: removal of the uterus via the vagina, thus avoiding an abdominal incision.

Varicose veins board: a wide board placed under the legs before surgery to allow for abduction and therefore better surgical access.

Vascular: appertaining to the blood vessels and blood supply.

Vasectomy: removal of a section of vas so that semen flow from the testes to the shaft of the penis is interrupted.

Viscera: organs within the body cavities; especially used to describe those of the abdomen, such as the stomach and intestines.

Index

205